The Energy Pathways in Our Body

Healing through Acupuncture and Acupressure

The Energy Pathways in Our Body

Healing Through Acupuncture and Acupressure

Rama Venkataraman
(M.D. Acupuncture)
Indian Academy of Acupuncture Science

Srikunj Sadbhavana Manch
New Delhi

Cataloging in Publication Data — DK
[Courtesy: D.K. Agencies (P) Ltd. <docinfo@dkagencies.com>]

Venkataraman, Rama, author.
The energy pathways in our body : healing through acupuncture and acupressure / Rama Venkataraman.
pages cm
Reprint. Originally published: 1996.
ISBN 9788182650183 (PB)

1. Acupuncture. 2. Acupressure. 3. Energy medicine. I. Title.

LCC RM184.V46 2026 | DDC 615.892 23

ISBN : 978-81-8265-018-3
First published in 1996
Second revised edition published in 2012
Reprinted in: 2019, 2023
Third reprint 2026

Published by:
Srikunj Sadbhavana Manch
"Srikunj", F-52, Bali Nagar
New Delhi - 110015

Distributed by:
D.K. Printworld (P) Ltd.
Regd. office : "Vedaśrī", F-395, Sudarshan Park
(Metro Station: ESI Hospital), New Delhi - 110015
Phones : (011) 4172 2626, 98713 94815
e-mail : indology@dkprintworld.com
Web : www.dkprintworld.com

I dedicate this book to
the divine power around us
which gave me the inspiration
to understand and spread
this subtle science
for the benefit of mankind.

Foreword

ACUPUNCTURE and acupressure are drugless therapies of Indian origin, now labelled as Chinese, because they received patronage in China. This is a simple, safe, economical and yet very effective form of treatment. It is very useful for prevention of diseases, for the *First Aid* treatment in case of acute emergencies and for treatment of many common ailments of day-to-day life. Understanding this information will help in giving relief to a wide range of health problems. Acupuncture/Acupressure, being economical, may prove to be a boon for the developing countries like India. Expenses for drugs may be curtailed to be used to fulfil the basic needs of the people.

Dr Rama Venkataraman is a noted acupuncture therapist. I am very happy that this student of mine has taken a lot of efforts to compile this book. I hope that this book will be very much useful for the learners of this science. I congratulate her for writing this book and wish her success in her future life.

Prof. Sir Dr P.B. Lohiya
Chairman, Indian Academy of Acupuncture Science

Preface

For the last few years, a sense of unease had entered in me, on seeing people around me becoming victims of bewildering kinds of ailments. Though many have the grit to grin and bear with the illness stoically, I could sense a total feeling of helplessness against ailments which play havoc to their quest for peaceful existence.

Many of the modern diseases are long-drawn, requiring life-long medication, like diabetes, high blood pressure or the crippling ones, like spondylosis, asthma or still worse the fatal ones like heart attack and many others. The treatment offered for most of the diseases are costly and time-consuming. Many of my near and dear ones were also victims to such ailments.

This led me to a long and determined search into the literature on alternative medicine. I pored over a wide variety of medical topics ranging from yoga, meditation, magnetic therapy, gem therapy, reflexology, acupressure, acupuncture, etc. My search was for a therapy which is effective, economical as well as easy to understand and follow.

When I came across the ancient therapy of acupuncture, more popularly followed in China and other Far East countries, I seemed to have found the answer to my search. The therapy appealed to me for a few reasons.

1. It is an effective, time-tested method and has an answer for a wide spectrum of diseases, from minor to major.
2. It can be easily understood by large number of people. With few explanatory lectures the person may be able to use it for any health problem.

3. It is most economical. It does not involve intake or use of any medication except the knowledge of right pressure points in the body.
4. It has absolutely no side effects. The therapy can be followed along with other medical disciplines like Allopathy, Homoeopathy, etc. Then the dosage of medicines can be decreased as stimulation of the points takes effect.

In the following pages I have explained as to how the therapy works, its concepts and practical applicability. The endeavour is to spread the wealth of this time-tested, effective medical knowledge to maximum number of people.

Dr Rama Venkataraman
e-mail: <ramavenkat75@gmail.com>
Website: <www.acupuncturebyrama.com>

Contents

1

Introduction

THE therapy as explained in the following pages has its base in the acupuncture principle. This is an ancient and effective medical therapy followed in the East for many centuries. As to the origin of the therapy it is still shrouded in debate. Though in the later years it found wide acceptability in China and Far East countries, its long practice in India cannot be ruled out. Some of the moxibustion and branding techniques followed in Kerala where "*Marmasthans*" are activated for the cure of different diseases have its origin in acupuncture therapy. But at the same time, while Chinese extensively developed it and penetrated the pressure points with needles for stimulation of the latent energy, in India over the course of time, with the development of Ayurveda and with current extensive stress on allopathy, these concepts neither developed further, nor did the existing knowledge receive science proper importance and due place.

However, knowledge, specifically health knowledge should not have any boundaries. Hence turning to the storehouse of knowledge as developed and practised by our neighbours, we can have a fresh insight into the dynamics of human body as per the concepts of this therapy.

Acupressure produces the same results as acupuncture when applied diligently. The location and understanding of these therapeutic points is more important for the effectiveness of the therapy. These points are found on the surface of the skin. They can be equated to small windows or openings facilitating the exchange of energy from the body to the outside cosmos and vice versa. The physical presence of these points was proved recently by Kirlian photography developed in Russia and Germany. This photography helps in taking photos of the energy around the body. The Kirlian photographs clearly brought to light the acupuncture points present in the body, which are the energy exchange points in the body.

Hence, it is very important to understand and use these energy points in the body and keep our body energy in harmony to remain in good health.

2

Understanding Acupuncture

ACUPUNCTURE is an ancient tested method for pain management as well as effective to treat variety of acute and chronic disorders.

Acupuncture treats the body in the energy level. Acupuncture points are found along the energy meridians running on the surface of the skin. Insertion of sterilised, fine filiform needles on the trigger points induces: **analgesic, immune enhancing, sedative, tranquillising** and **balancing reactions** in the body altering the body's metabolism and chemistry towards positive health.

The fact that stimulation of these trigger points brings out anaesthetic effect and major operations are conducted in other parts of the world proves the pain-removing effect of acupuncture beyond doubt.

It is almost a painless therapy. The needle prick can be only as painful as an ant bite.

Acupuncture can also serve as an effective companion and act as complementary to other modern methods of treatment. It can be a very effective and valuable orthopaedic tool. In many unrecognised pains, which defy diagnosis, like backache, joint pains, post-operative trauma, hand and leg pain, non-healing fractures, motor recovery, etc. it can give hope and speedy recovery.

Needling

Acupuncture needling is a relatively painless procedure. The needles are of very thin gauge, almost, like a wire. It is easy to administer. **The use of individual needles for each patient removes the risk of any contamination**. The efffectiveness of needling is proved beyond any doubt.

Effects of Acupuncture

By inserting needle at the correct trigger point remarkable changes are brought in the body. Some are physical and some are chemical. While physical changes are subjectively felt by the patient, many chemical changes can be empirically recorded.

CHEMICAL EFFECTS

It has been scientifically tested and proved the following changes happen in the chemistry of the body after acupuncture.

Immunity Improving

Increase in

1. White blood corpuscles (leucocytes)
2. Antibodies
3. Red blood corpuscles
4. Gamma globulins

Pain Recovery

Increase in

1. Endorphins
2. Encephaline
3. Numerous Neurotransmitters

Neurological

1. Dopamine content of the brain

Sedative

1. Delta and theta wave activity

Circulatory

Decrease in

1. The blood clots

PHYSICAL EFFECTS

A sense of well-being spreads in the body soon after administrating the acupuncture. As the therapy works on energy level the patient feels energetic and active. Thus it is felt the therapy adds life to years making the person more alive.

The noticeable effects are:

1. Relaxation
2. Tonification of the body
3. Pain removal
4. Motor recovery (improves movement)
5. Immunity improving (decrease in infection)
6. Balancing (decrease in blood pressure and balance of hormone, endocrine and enzyme secretions)
7. A sense of well-being both physical and mental (psychological)

Acupressure of Acupuncture Points

For purpose of self-administration acupressure of acupuncture points is one of the simplest, economical and easily acceptable methods of treatment. When employed with care and consistency, **acupressure can prove to be an equally effective tool of treatment.**

Some of the techniques of acupressure to be employed in the energy meridian pathways are discussed below:

First one should understand the direction of energy moving in the meridian selected for treatment.

Energy moves in the meridian in two ways:

1. Towards the head, and
2. Towards the fingers or toes.

The energy increases — if pressure is given along the flow of the meridian. **Helps in tonifying.**

Decrease if pressure is given against the flow of the meridian. **Helps in sedating.**

Techniques of Using Pressure Instruments

1. By hand — Fingers, palm, wrist, elbow can be used.
2. By a blunt object — Wooden rod, metal rod called jimmy or even toothpick or matchstick can be used.
3. By a small table tennis ball — The rounded surface is an effective and acceptable surface for giving pressure. Rounded vegetable like lemon, gooseberry, small potatoes can also be used.
4. Small and big rollers.

Anatomy of Pressure Points

The acupressure/acupuncture points are small, pin-sized openings lying on the surface of skin along the pathway of energy meridian. As they are two-way entry for energy, the energy can be either pushed into the meridian or drawn out.

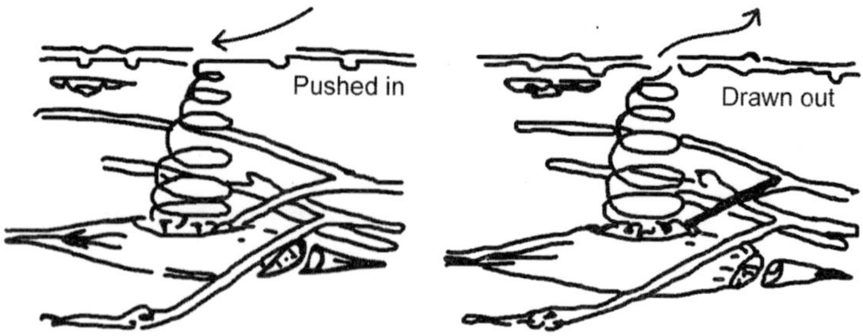

Check for Deficiency or Excess

Since the treatment is given in energy level it is important to determine the condition of energy in the body and the pertaining meridian/organ to be treated. The energy can be deficient, excess or normal.

Ways to Determine

Deficiency — Cool skin and pain on light pressure indicates deficiency. There can be lassitude, weakness, feeling for taking rest. **It is an yin state**.

Excess — Hot skin, pain on heavy pressure indicates excess. Sharp pains are associated with excess energy. **It is a yang state**.

Normal — Elastic firm skin indicates normal flow of energy.

Pressure-Applying Methods

To stimulate — If the energy is deficient it has to be increased or tonified.

Pressure can be given —

1. In pumping motion.
2. Clockwise rotatory motion along the flow of meridian.

The pressure can be given either with finger pressure, jimmy with a rounded ball.

To Sedate — If the energy is excess it has to decreased.

Pressure can be given —

Anticlockwise in a rotatory motion against flow of the meridian. The pressure can be given either with finger pressure, jimmy or with a rounded ball.

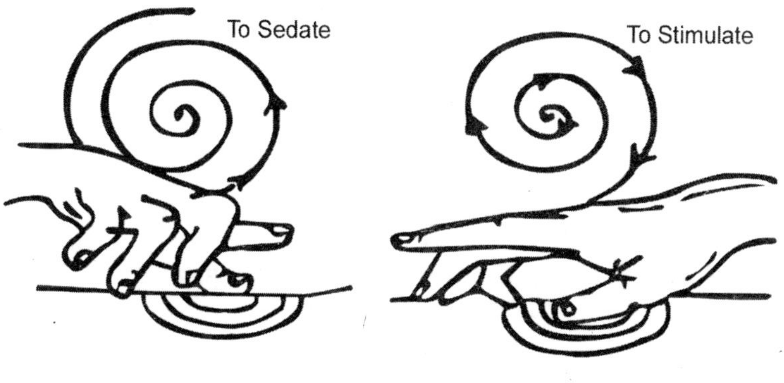

Duration

The pressure should be given as per the problem.

Some General Rules Are:

1. Pressure should be given in each point or along a single meridian for one or two minutes.
2. The pressure can be repeated twice or thrice a day like taking a dose of medicine.
3. Dont't give pressure in full stomach or in famished state.
4. The pressure should be given in a comfortable, tolerable way.
5. Tender spots should be pressed gently and consistently over a period of time.

Treating Pressure Points by Hand

1. **Acupressure** — The points are given pressure with fingers, knuckles, elbow, fist or palm. This helps in stimulation of the points.
2. **Pinching** — As the points lay on the surface of the skin, pinching can be an effective method to treat especially on soft portion like face, belly, forearm where the bone structure is not strong to apply pressure.

   Pinching pressure can also be given on the ends of fingers where many of the meridians start and end and the energy is very active and mobile.
3. **Rubbing** — This helps in increasing friction and flow of energy.
4. **Tapping and Pounding** — The points and the meridian can also be tapped with finger tips or pounded with knuckles and wrist bone to activate and stimulate.
5. **Massage** — It is an age-old technique which helps in rejuvenating the energy flow. There are many methods of massage. However, while doing meridian massage it has

to be kept in mind, that if the objective is to stimulate or sedate; accordingly it should be done against the meridian (sedate) or towards the flow of meridian (tonify).

Pressure Points by Hand

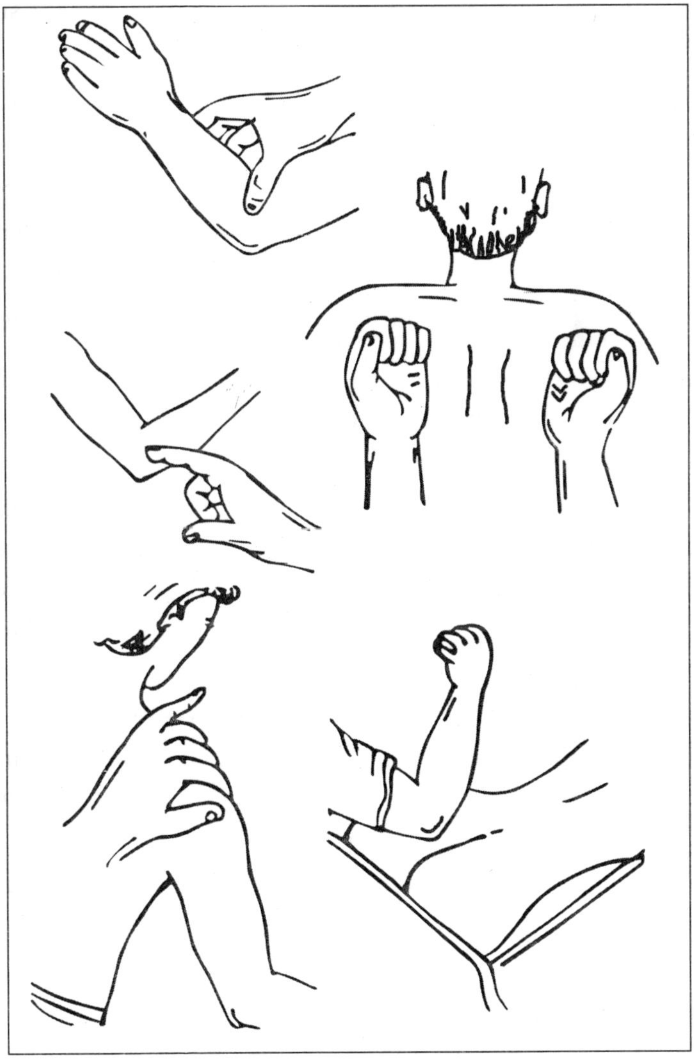

Other Methods of Stimulation

Moxibustion — In this method heat is applied on pressure points with dried leaves of moxa plants. Heat can also be applied by incense sticks — *agarbattis* — if moxa is not available. It is useful for arthritic conditions.

Cryopuncture — In case of inflammation or burning sensation, ice packs can be applied in pressure points.

Magnet Acupuncture — Small button magnets are fixed over the pressure points by tape.

The principle: North Pole — Tonifies, South Pole — Sedates

Seed Stimulation — Seed of commonly used plants like *channa, soya, moong* and mustard are taped over pressure points and pressed periodically. The natural energy present in the seeds will help to stimulate the points.

Tapping with Needless — Tapping the pressure points with needles along the meridian path and applying heat/moxa can help in increasing the energy flow.

Laser Therapy — Mild lasers made of Helium-Neon can be safely used to stimulate the points.

Colour Beads — Colour therapy can be applied to treat the points with colour beads.

Red and Yellow	—	For stimulation
Black and Dark Blue	—	For sedation
Pink, Violet, Green	—	For neutral effect

The colour beads can be taped on points and pressed periodically.

There are other methods like sonopuncture, cupping, transcutaneous electrical stimulation, catgut embedding, press needle embedding, etc. However, these will require clinical help.

Other Methods of Stimulation

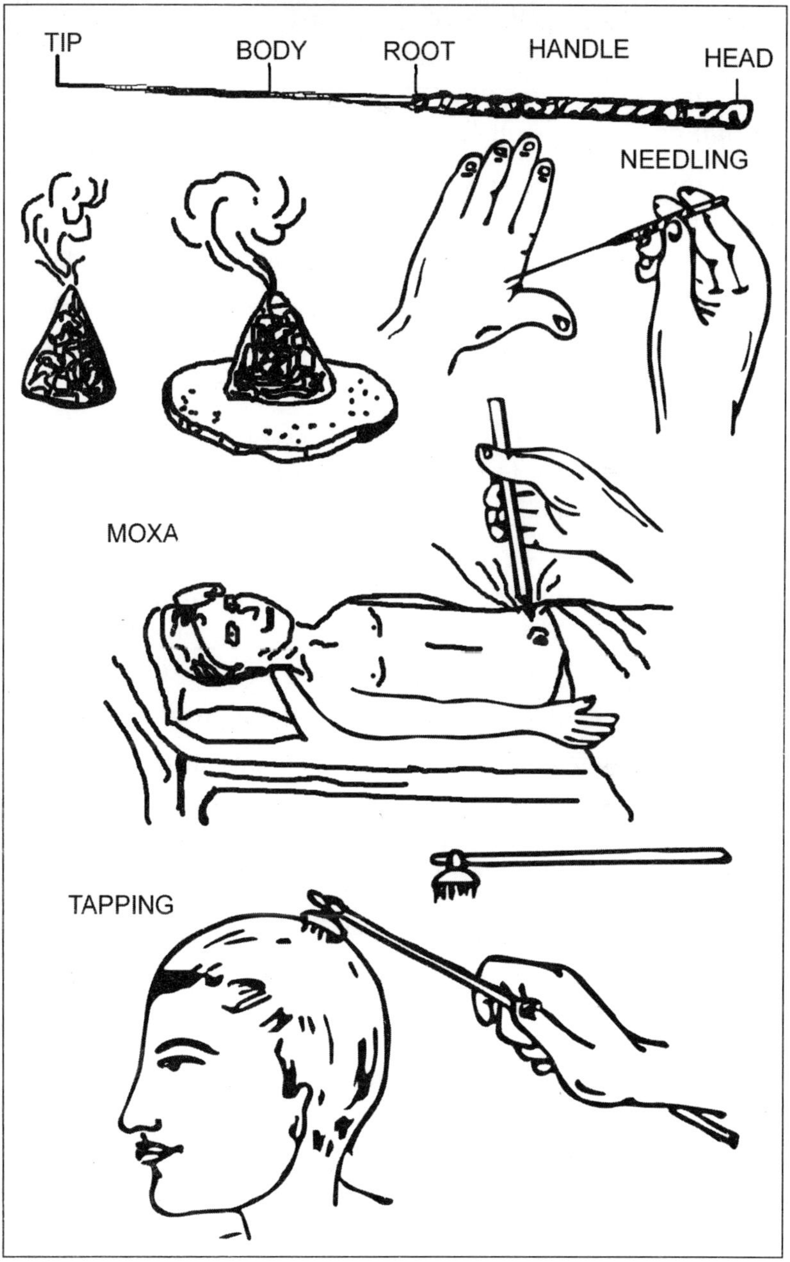

Facial Pressure Points

It is said that face is the index of a person. The statement is also true by pressure methods. There are number of give away points in the face which can be used both for diagnosing and treatment of vital organs of our body.

Large Intestine 20 — The ending point of large intestine lies 0.5 chun next to flair of the nose. Pinching this point helps in deducing the condition of large intestine.

Stomach 1, 2, 3, 4 — They lie in a line below the pupil of the eye. They are the starting points of stomach meridian. Help in knowing stomach meridian and stomach condition.

Small Intestine (S.I.) 18 & 19 — S.I. 18 lies on the cheekbone and S.I. 19 lies close to ear at the end of the cheek. This is the ending point of small intestine. It helps to deduce the condition of small intestine.

Gall Bladder (G.B.) 1 & 2 — G.B. 1 lies at the end of the outer canthus of the eye 0.5 chun below and G.B. 2 lies in front of tragus of the ear. They are the starting points of gall bladder channel. They help in finding out the condition of gall bladder.

Urinary Bladder (U.B.) 1 & 2 — U.B. 1 lies in front of inner canthus of the eye and U.B. 2 lies in the tip of the eyebrow above U.B. 1. They are the starting points of urinary bladder. They help in deducing the condition of urinary bladder.

Triple Heater (T.H.) 21 & 23 — T.H. 21 lies in front of the ears. T.H. 23 at the tip of the eyebrow. These are the ending points of triple heater. They reveal the state of triple heater channel in the body.

Governing Meridian (DU) 25 & 26 — DU 25 is found at the tip of nose and DU 26, 0.5 chun above the lips. They are ending points of the ruling meridian of the yang channels. They are the indicators of the brain activity and status of yang meridians.

Facial Pressure Points

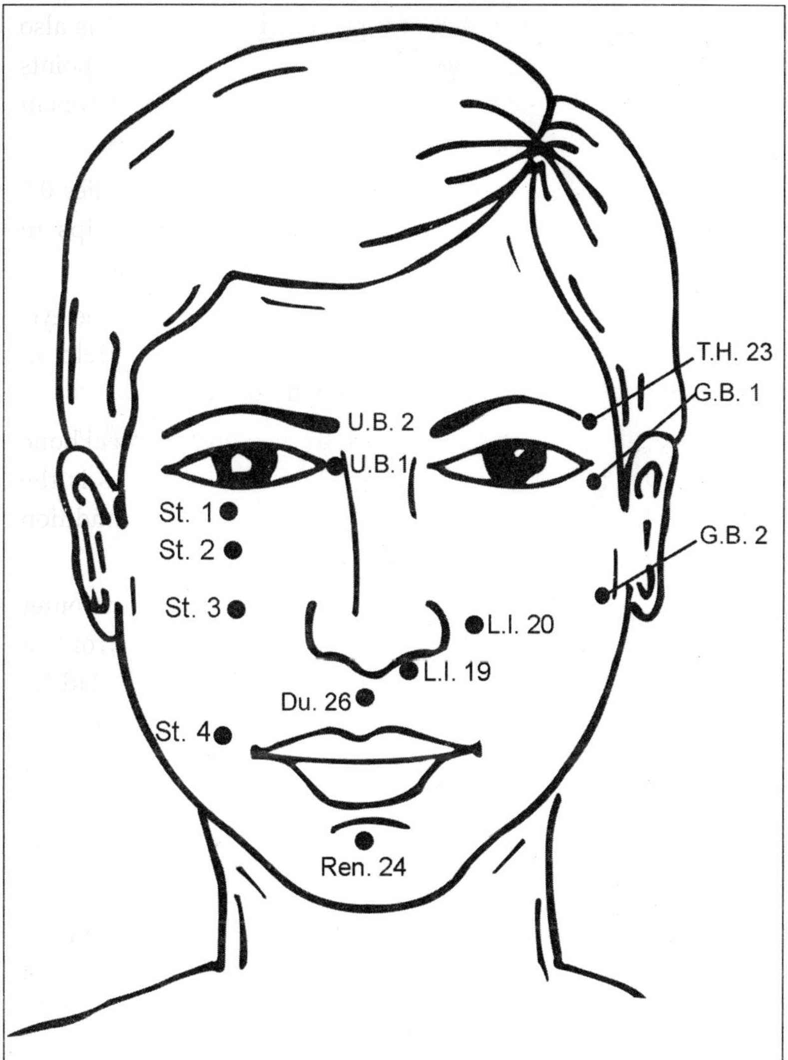

Conception Vessel (Ren) 24 — It is found on the chin. It is ending point of ruling meridian of yin channels. It indicates the states of yin channels.

As these points are either starting or ending points of the meridian, the energy found here is very active and mobile. The

Facial Pressure Points

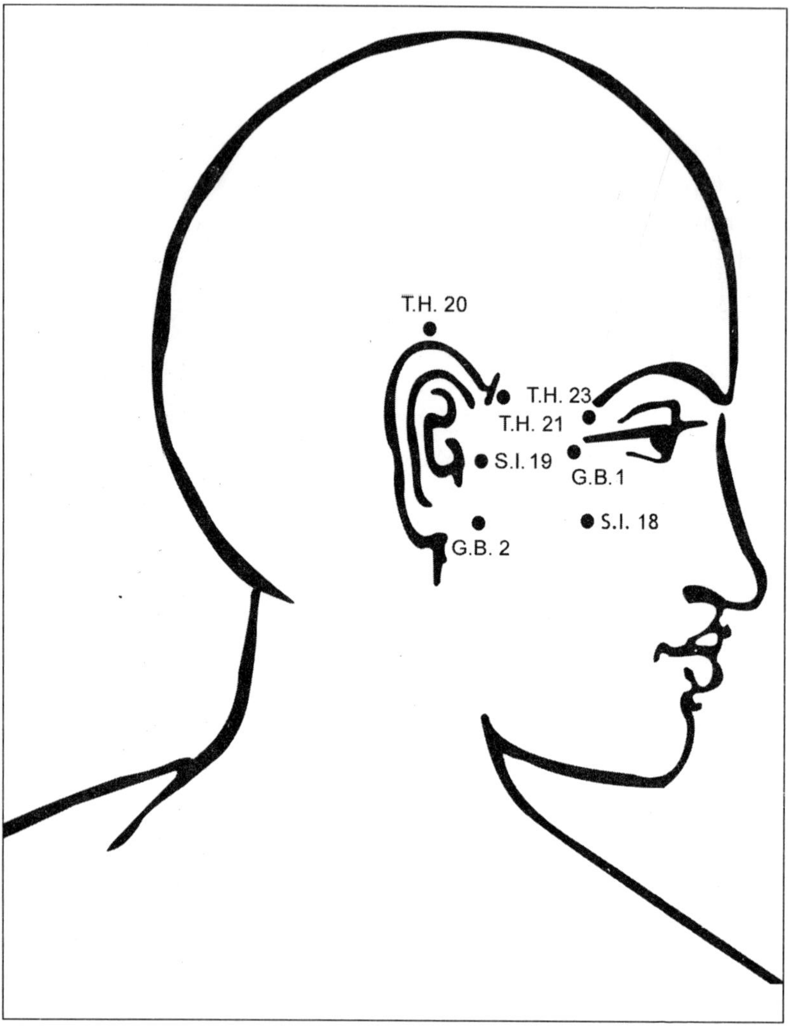

points can be used for testing and treatment. Any pain in these points either on light pressure or heavy pressure indicates disturbance of the meridian and the pertaining organ.

They can be checked up every morning. Activated by pinching and pressure if they are found limp, or can be sedated by dispersing the energy doing anticlockwise rotations.

Alarm Points

The remarkable feature of this science is, each of the organs issuing an energy meridian has two alarm points indicating the condition of the organ. Their position has been shown below.

When the working of a vital organ is disturbed, the corresponding alarm point becomes tender. Each organ has two alarm points, one on the front side and another on the back side of the body.

Organ	Alarm Points	
	Front	Back
Lung	Lu. 1	U.B. 13
Pericardium	Ren. 17	U.B. 14
Heart	Ren. 14	U.B. 15
Liver	Liv. 14	U.B. 18
Gall bladder	G.B. 24	U.B. 19
Spleen	Liv. 13	U.B. 20
Stomach	Ren. 12	U.B. 21
Triple heater	Ren. 5	U.B. 22
Kidney	G.B. 25	U.B. 23
Large intestine	St. 25	U.B. 25
Small intestine	Ren. 4	U.B. 27
Urinary baldder	Ren. 3	U.B. 28

Front Alarm Points

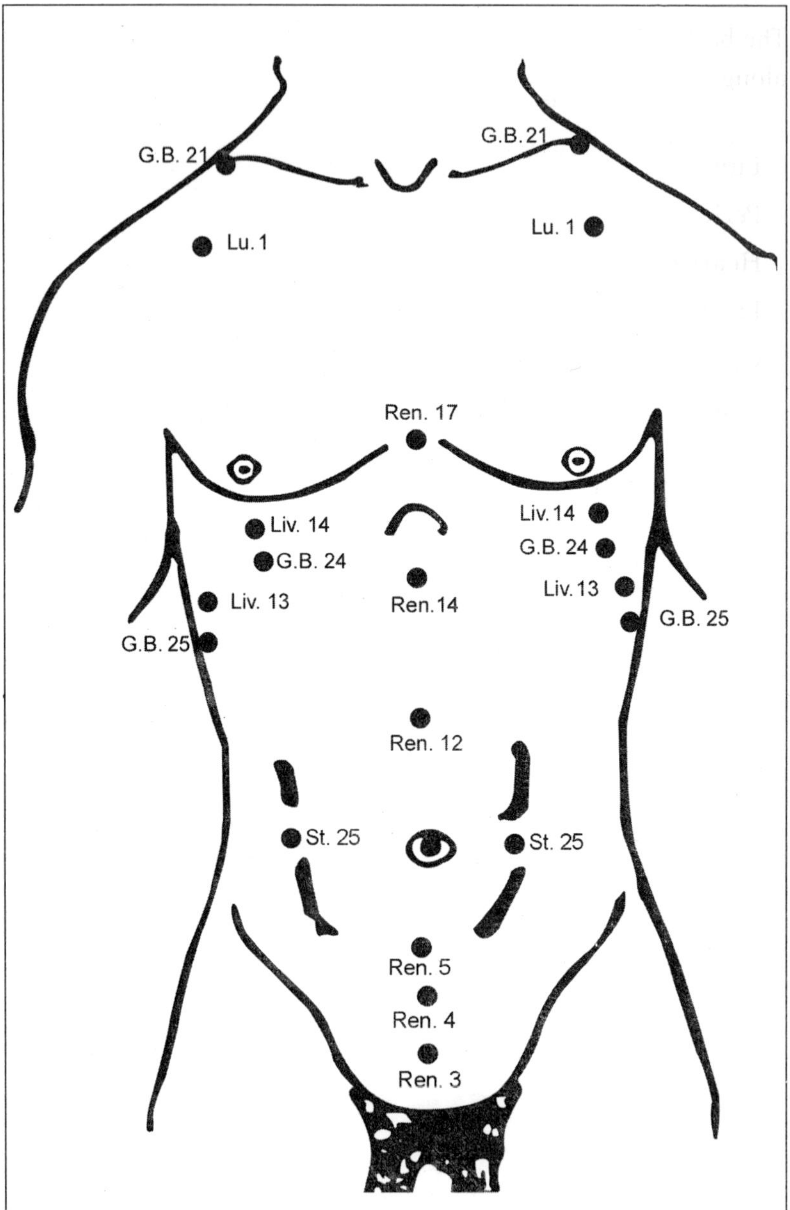

Note: The special point of the Gall Bladder at the shoulder is also included.

The Back Alarm Points

The back alarm points lie 1.5 chun lateral to the vertebral column along the lower border of each vertebra.

Back Alarm Points

Lung	—	U.B. 13	Stomach	—	U.B. 21
Pericardium	—	U.B. 14	Triple heater	—	U.B. 22
Heart	—	U.B. 15	Kidney	—	U.B. 23
Liver	—	U.B. 18	Large intestine	—	U.B. 25
Gall bladder	—	U.B. 19	Small intestine	—	U.B. 27
Spleen	—	U.B. 20	Urinary bladder	—	U.B. 28

The Back Alarm Points

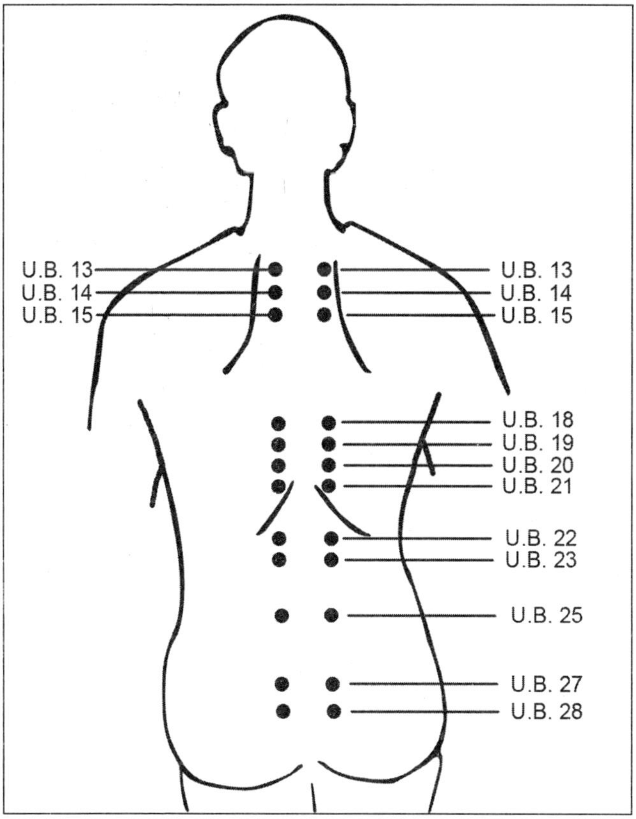

Special Alarm Points

These are four of them. These points also help in diagnosis.

1. Liver disorder — Liv. 6
2. Gall bladder disorder — G.B. 21
3. Vermiform appendix — Ex 33 (Extraordinary point 33), 2 chun below St. 36.
4. Gall bladder and Liver disorder — Ex. 35, 1 chun below G.B. 34.

Special Alarm Points

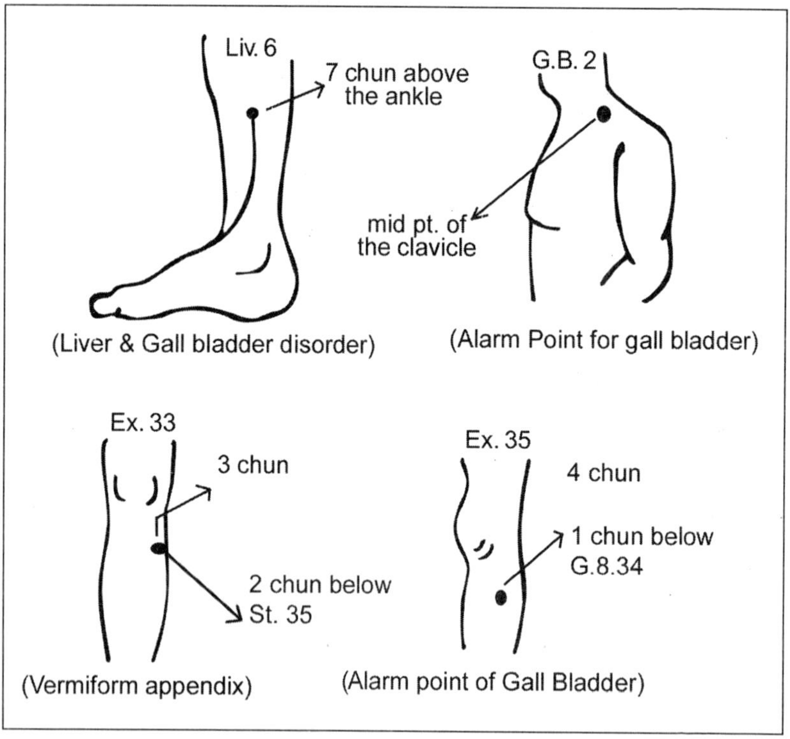

These alarm points help not only in diagnosis but also in therapy. When the disease condition improves the alarm points become less tender.

Improving the Working of Vital Organs

Apart from this there are also certain vital points lying along the pathway of the meridian, which help to diagnose and treat a particular organ.

Lungs — Squeeze the outer side of the thumb to know the status of lungs. Sharp pain indicates functioning disturbed.

Heart — Squeeze the inner side of the little finger to activate the heart. Give pressure on the palm below little finger as shown in *fig*. to get a boost of energy from heart.

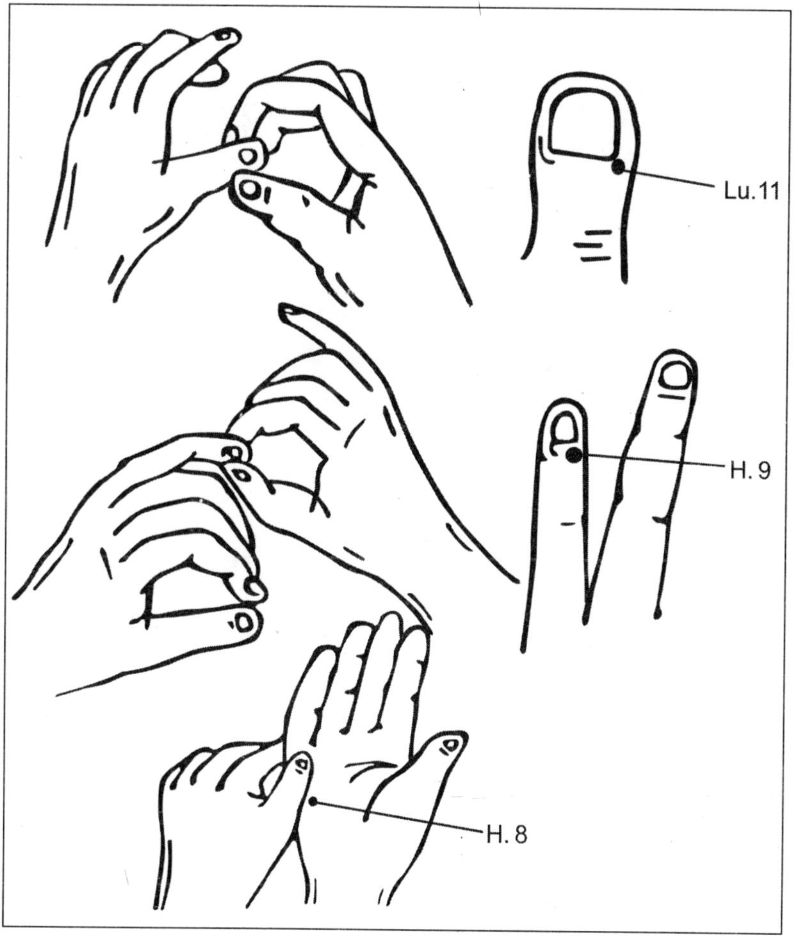

Liver — Deep pressure two fingers away between the web of 1st and 2nd toes improves the working of liver and avoids hepatic condition.

Liver and Gall Bladder — Firm pressure by knuckles below the breast in line with the nipples improves liver and gall bladder working.

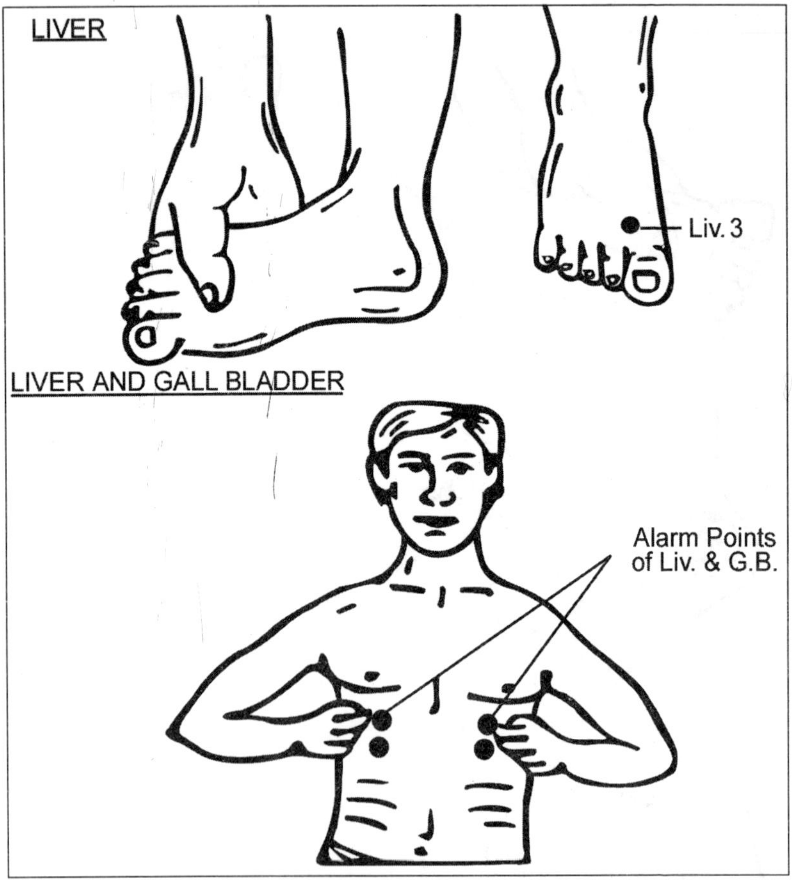

Kidney — Apply firm pressure on the depression of the upper 1/3rd part of the foot. Kidney meridian starts there and it gives a boost to the working of kidney.

Also take a small ball and apply rotatory pressure around the ankles both inside and outside to improve the working of **sexglands** connected with kidney.

Spleen — To activate spleen keep a finger at the outer end of the first toe and squeeze it firmly. Apply a moxa or incense stick to pass energy into the channel. Spleen takes care of your allergy and immunity problems.

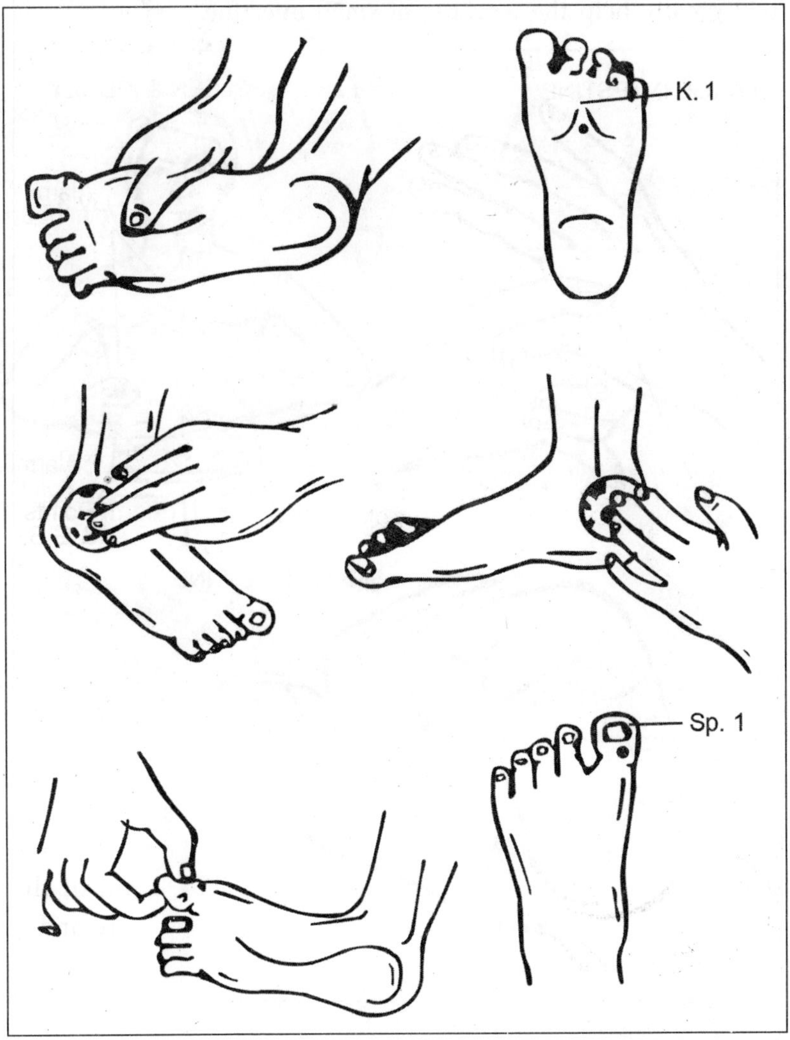

Spleen and Kidney — They can be together activated by applying knuckle pressure in the waist region pointing towards the front side. The alarm points of kidney and spleen lie there.

Large Intestine — To activate an insipid and constipated colon, give firm pressure at L.I. 4 as shown.

Small Intestine — Pinch and squeeze the side of the palm along the little finger where the front and the back sides meet. It will greatly help the working of small intestine.

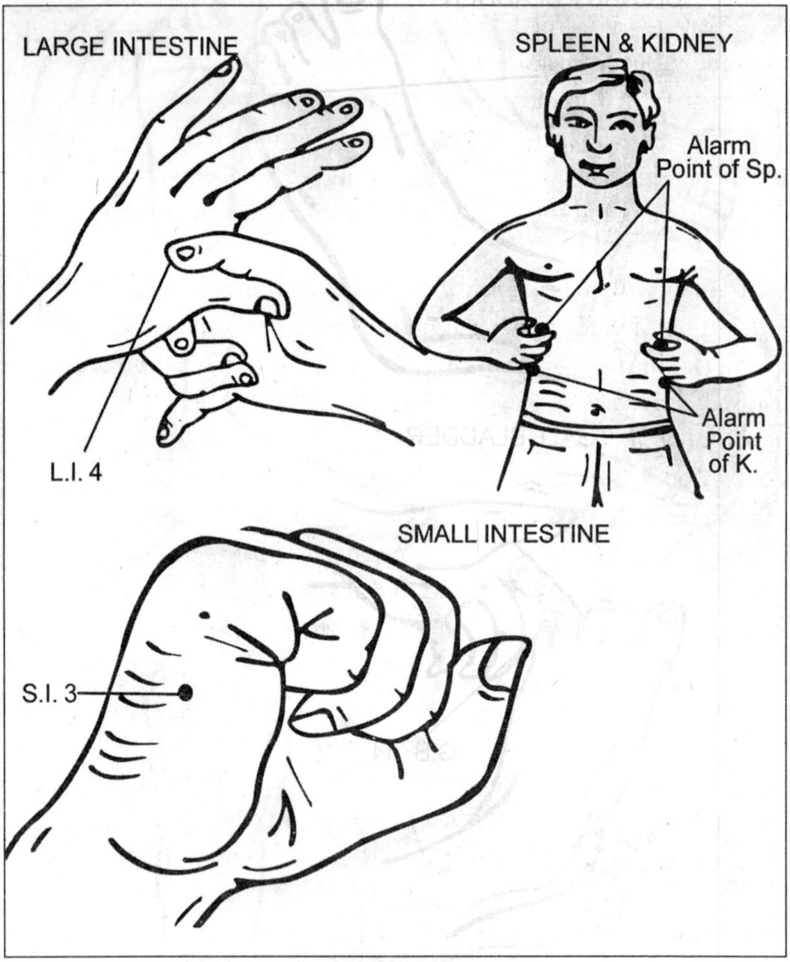

Urinary Bladder — Squeeze the little toe vigorously and also rotate a ball on the outer side of the ankle. You will be surprised to find apart from the bladder improving in function your backache also takes leave of you.

Gall Bladder — Squeeze the 4th toe, which is the end point of gall bladder and rotate a ball over the dorsum of foot between the 4th and 5th toes to activate the organ.

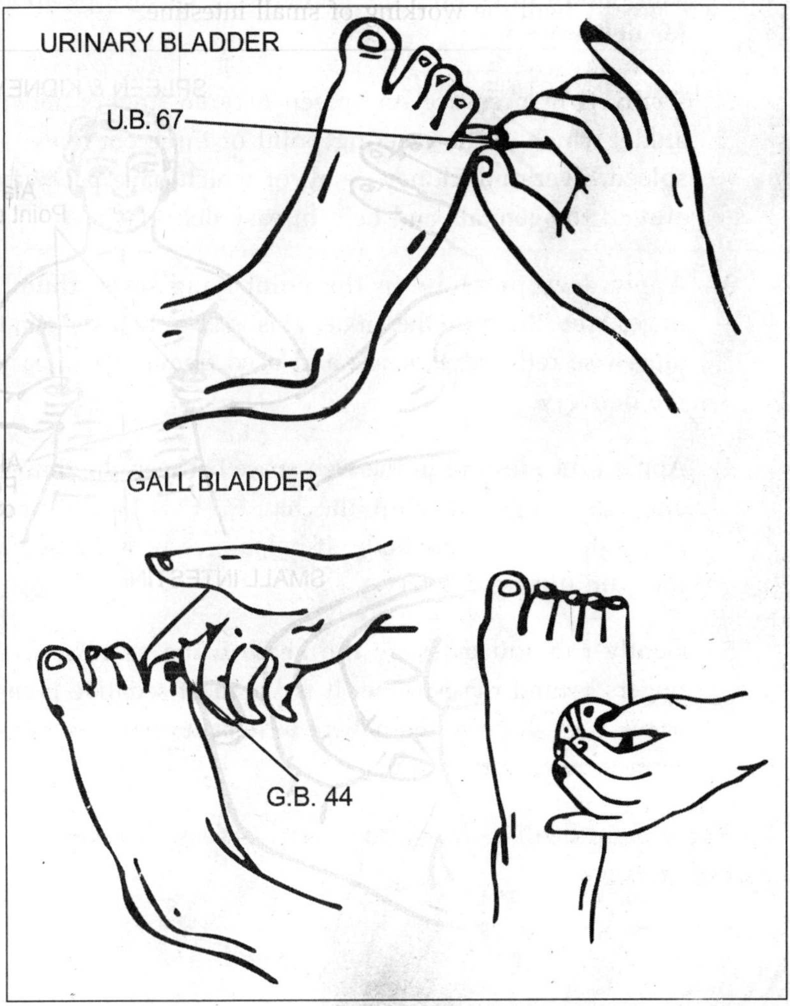

Easy Delivery

Acupuncture science has been used from time immemorial as an aid for easy and painless delivery.

1. Apply moxa or heat at the tip of little finger. It is U.B. 67 point which goes up till the pelvis and above. Activating this point helps in easy movement of pelvis and many times helps in turning the foetus to face down position for delivery.

2. Apply firm pressure on spleen 6 three fingers above ankle, which is the meeting point of three energies — spleen, liver and kidney — all of which have pathway around the genitals and help in easy delivery.

3. Apply deep pressure on the point lying seven thumb finger breadth above the ankle. This is also the liver point otherwise referred as *neima* and used frequently to ease the delivery.

4. Apply firm pressure in the web space between the thumb and first finger in both the hands. This is the best analgesic point in the body. It helps greatly in reducing the pain during delivery.

5. Gently rub and massage the head in the middle, five fingers behind the hairline. It is the most sedative point of the body. It helps the patient to remain calm and saves from unnecessary trauma.

These points will without fail assure an easy, smooth and normal delivery.

Easy Delivery

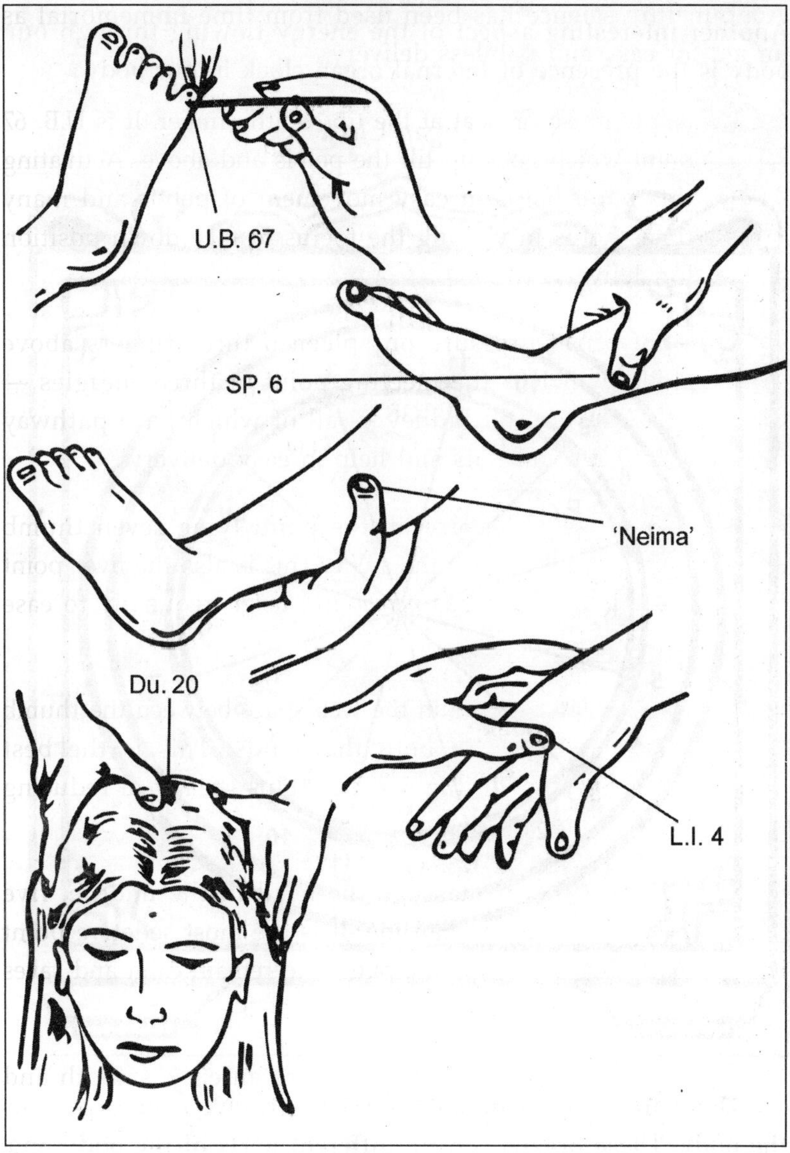

Organ Clock

Another interesting aspect of the energy flowing through our body is the presence of internal organ clock in our body.

Organ Clock

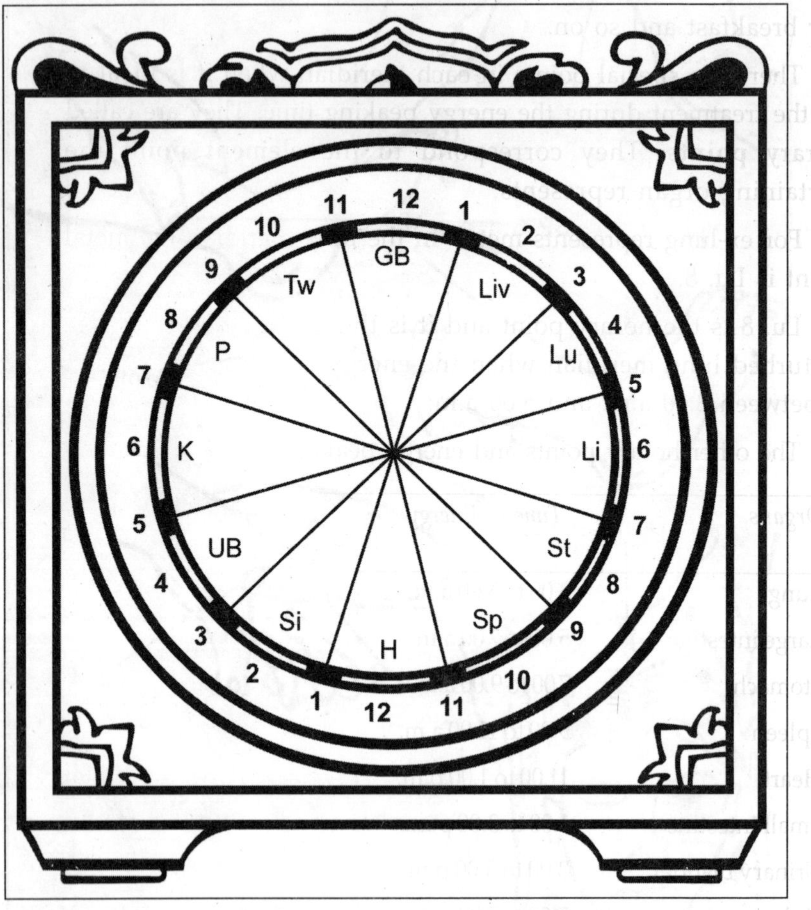

There are as per acupuncture science twelve main organs in the body. These organs control different parts of the body and sense organs.

It is found the energy peaks in each organ for two hours in 24-hour period of the day completing a day's cycle.

The organ clock below shows the peak energy time of each pertaining organ.

Thus we see 5.00 a.m. to 7.00 a.m. when large intestine energy peaks and we pass stools.

And 7.00 a.m. to 9.00 a.m. when stomach peaks and we have our breakfast and so on.

There are special points in each meridian when it is ideal to do the treatment during the energy peaking time. They are called **horary points**. They correspond to the element point the pertaining organ represents.

For ex-lung represents metal. In the lung meridian the metal point is Lu. 8.

Lu. 8 is the horary point and it is the best point to treat the disturbed lung meridian when the energy peaks in that, which is between 3.00 a.m. and 5.00 a.m.

The other horary points and energy peaking time are as under:

Organs	*Time of Energy*	*Horary Points (Treatment Points)*
Lung	3.00 to 5.00 a.m.	Lu. 8
Large intestine	5.00 to 7.00 a.m.	L.I. 1
Stomach	7.00 to 9.00 a.m.	St. 36
Spleen	9.00 to 11.00 a.m.	Sp. 3
Heart	11.00 to 1.00 p.m.	H. 8
Small intestine	1.00 to 3.00 p.m.	S.I. 5
Urinary bladder	3.00 to 5.00 p.m.	U.B. 66
Kidney	5.00 to 7.00 p.m.	K. 10
Pericardium	7.00 to 9.00 p.m.	P. 8
Triple Heater	9.00 to 11.00 p.m.	T.H. 6
Gall bladder	11.00 to 1.00 p.m.	G.B. 41
Liver	1.00 to 3.00 p.m.	Liv. 1

3

Concept

THE theory of Yin and Yang forms the basis of acupuncture.

Yin and Yang are the two opposite forces present in the body. As a result of interaction of these forces "Qi" or *Prana,* the vital energy is created. Yin is considered the negative or female force and Yang is considered the positive or male force. These forces are constantly interacting with one another. A balance between these forces keeps the body in a healthy state. An imbalance creates disease.

As per the Chinese therapy, the Yin and Yang forces are all-pervading in the universe. Man is a microcosm in the universe. His energies constantly interchange with the energies of the macrocosm, the universe. Thus there is a constant inflow and out-flow of energy. An excess or deficiency in Yin and Yang causes imbalance in "Qi" the vital energy. The basic concept of acupuncture is hence the balancing of energies in the body and bring it to a harmonious level with the outside energy.

When	Yin	=	Yang	indicates healthy state.
	Yin	#	Yang	leads to disease.
	Yin	>	Yang	causes deficiency.
	Yin	<	Yang	causes excess
	Yang	=	0	leads to death
	Yin	=	infinity	

4

Cause of Diseases

DISEASES are caused by two factors.

1. Exogenous factors (External factors) — Like wind, cold, heat, humidity, dryness, fire.

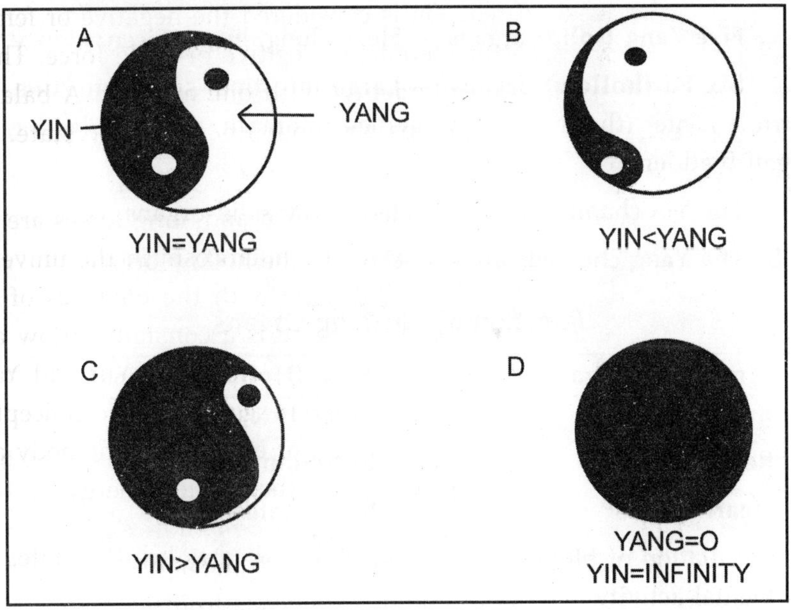

2. Endogenous factors (Internal Factors) — Like joy, anger, melancholy, obsession sorrow, horror, surprise, shock.

Any disturbance in these affects the balance of "Qi" the vital energy in the pertaining organ. While in exogenous factors the channels are first disturbed then the internal organ gets affected, in the endogenous factors the internal organ gets affected, then the effect reaches the channel.

5

Organs of the Body

THE solid organs of the body are called the **Zang organs.**

The hollow organs of the body are called the **Fu organs.**

The important organs which the therapy recognises are:

Five Zang (solid) organs — Heart, lung, liver, spleen, kidney.

Six Fu (hollow) organs — Large intestine, small intestine, triple heater (the three body cavities), stomach, urinary bladder, gall bladder.

The Yin channels are connected to the solid organs.

The Yang channels are connected to the hollow organs.

Function of Yin-Yang Organs

Yin (Solid Organs)	Yang (Hollow Organs)
Lung	**Large Intestine**
Respiration	Excretion
Heart	**Small Intestine**
Circulation of blood, mental activity	Separation of essence
Pericardium	**Triple Heater**
Same as the heart	Houses the organs, balances the triple cavities
Spleen	**Stomach**
Water metabolism, immunity, circulation of blood	Digestion, transport of the food and water

Liver	**Gall Bladder**
Storage and transport of blood, regulates muscles, tendons, endocrines	Storage of bile, mental activity
Kidney	**Urinary Bladder**
Regulates blood pressure, bone, cartilage, teeth, nail, head hair, genital activity	Water balance, genital balance

The Meridians

The Yin and Yang energies flow through certain routes in the body. The course of this route is called meridians or channels.

There are six pairs of Yin channels in the body, six pairs of Yang channels and two individual channels formed by joining the extra points which lie in a line.

They are called governing meridian (Du channel) and conception meridian (Ren channel).

Thus there are in all fourteen meridians traversing along the body surface. Of these twelve are in pair, two are single.

The Names of the Fourteen Meridians

Lung meridian, pericardium meridian, heart meridian.	3 Yin channels of the hand
Spleen meridian, liver meridian, kidney meridian.	3 Yin channels of the leg
Large intestine meridian, triple heater meridian, small intestine meridian.	3 Yang channels of the hand
Stomach meridian, gall bladder, urinary bladder meridian.	3 Yang channels of the leg

Channels Governing other Meridians

Governing vessel meridian
(Du channel)

Conception vessel meridian
(Ren channel)

The Yin channels lie along the front side of the body. They are connected to the solid organs like lung, liver, spleen, kidney, heart, etc.

The Yang channels lie along the outer side of the body. They are connected to the hollow organs like stomach, gall bladder, intestines, urinary bladder, etc.

The Route

The energy in these channels takes the following route.

3 Yin channels of the hand start from chest → flow to the palm
(meet the 3 Yang channels of the hand near the nail)

3 Yang channels of the hand start from the palm → flow to the head
(meet the 3 Yang channels of the foot)

3 Yang channels of the leg start from the head → flow to the foot
(meet the 3 Yin channels of the foot)

3 Yin channels of the leg start from the foot → flow to the chest
(meet the 3 Yin channels of the hand)

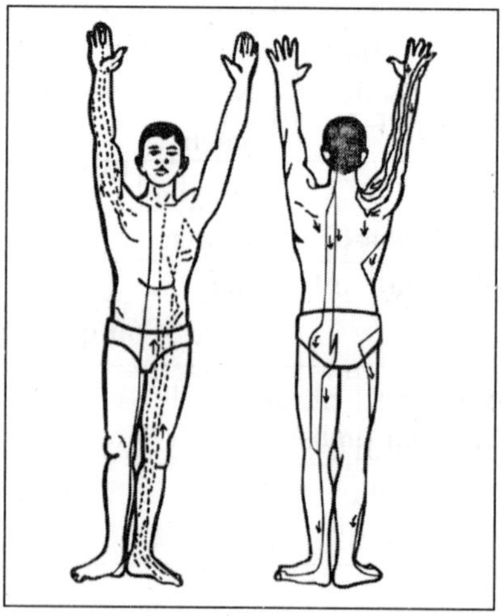

When a man stands, with arms raised, the Yang energy descends from the hand to the foot along the outer side, while the Yin energy ascends along the inner side from the foot towards the chest and hand completing the energy cycle.

The Yin-Yang Connections

Each of the Yin channels is connected to a Yang channel.

This forms six pairs of connection. They are:

Lung channel	Connected to	Large intestine channel
Pericardium channel	Connected to	Triple heater channel
Heart channel	Connected to	Small intestine channel
Liver channel	Connected to	Gall bladder channel
Spleen channel	Connected to	Stomach channel
Kidney channel	Connected to	Urinary bladder channel

Each of the Yin organs and the corresponding Yin meridians is connected to a tissue and a sense organ as well as to a Yang meridian. Thus a pair of Yin, Yang meridian **influences the working of the connected tissue and sense organs.**

The Chart Showing Yin-yang Connections to Different Tissues and Sense Organs

Yin organ	*Yang organ*	*Connecting tissue*	*Connecting sense organ*	*Connecting organ part for colour*	*Colour change*
Lu.	L.I.	Skin & Body hair	Nose smell	Skin	White
H.	S.I.	Brain & Blood vessel	Tongue speech	Mouth	Red
Liv.	G.B.	Muscle & Tendon	Eyes Sight	Nail	Green
Sp.	St.	Soft tissue (The four limbs)	Mouth taste	Lip	Yellow
K.	U.B.	Bone, teeth, head hair	Ear hearing	Inside of Forearm	Black

Yin organ	*Yang organ*	*Secretion*	*Emotion*	*Taste*	*Sound*
Lu.	L.I.	Mucous	Sadness	Pungent	Sobbing
H.	S.I.	Sweat	Joy	Bitter	Laughing
Liv.	G.B.	Tears	Anger	Sour	Shouting
Sp.	St.	Saliva	Obsession	Sweet	Singing
K.	U.B.	Urine	Fear	Salty	Groaning

Any disturbance in the organ is reflected in the corresponding tissue, sense organ, secretion, emotion, taste and sound.

6

Energy Points

THE energy in these meridians orginate from important organs of the body and then take peripheral superficial routes, close to the skin. It can be traced at this level, and the flow of energy along the superficial pathways can be modulated through sensitive points along these channels.

These sensitive points are the acupuncture points. These points tend to be tender, more painful than the rest of the parts and electrically have a low resistance and high conductivity.

They are bioelectrically active points and can be compared to a transformer in an electrical circuit which can step up and step down the energy flow as required.

Functions

INFLUENCE THE VITAL ORGANS

By applying pressure to these points the vital organ to which the channel is connected can be reached and its function rectified.

ACT AS DIAGNOSING AND TREATMENT POINTS

They are diagnosing as well as treatment points. Pain in the pressure points indicates a problem, the same can be rectified by applying pressure at the acupressure points.

ACT AS MOTOR POINTS

These points also act as motor points by helping the functioning of those parts over which a particular meridian runs.

Example: Stomach meridian has a long route, starting below the eye it travels over the face, neck, throat, abdomen, thigh, leg and ends up between 2nd and 3rd toes.

It hence has influence over the various organs like eyes, teeth, chest, stomach, leg muscles, etc.

INFLUENCE THE CONNECTED SENSE ORGANS AND TISSUE

Each meridian is connected to a sense organ and tissue.

Example : Lung channel is connected to

Sense organ — Nose

Tissue — Skin

Some pressure points in the lung channel are activated for skin ailments and nose related problems.

SPECIALISED THERAPEUTIC EFFECTS

Some pressure points produce particular therapeutic effects in the body.

They are **analgesic, sedative, homoeostatic, immune enhancing, psychological, motor recovery** and **tonification**. Hence stimulating these points act in recovering from the related setbacks.

Example : An analgesic reaction helps in alleviating pain like toothache, headache, pain of arthritis, low backache, etc.

Location of Energy Points

1. **By Anatomical Landmarks:** When points are present close to important known anatomical parts, it can be located easily.

   Example: L.I. 11 - The best homoeostatic point is located at the crease of the elbow joint along outer side.

2. **Tender Spots:** The energy points, especially the ones affected will be tender and painful, and thus can be located easily.

3. **Electronic Point Detector:** The meridians are bioelectric pathways. The energy points have lower resistance and higher electrical conductivity. This factor makes it easy to locate the points with an electronic instrument.

Chun Measurement

The unit of measurement is called a chun.

1 chun = Breadth of the thumb at its widest part.

1.5 chun = Combined breadth of middle finger and index finger.

Chun measurement of each person is according to the size of his/her finger and it varies from person to person.

Chunometer — It is an instrument, basically a caliper to measure chun. With this on measuring one unit, multiples of the same can be obtained.

Distance Between Some Important Anatomical Landmarks

Armpit crease to elbow crease	—	9 chun.
Elbow crease to wrist crease	—	12 chun.
Thigh to knee crease	—	19 chun.
Middle of knee crease to ankle crease	—	16 chun.
Navel to pubic border	—	5 chun.
Between two nipples	—	8 chun.
Two ribs	—	1 chun.

Chun Measurement

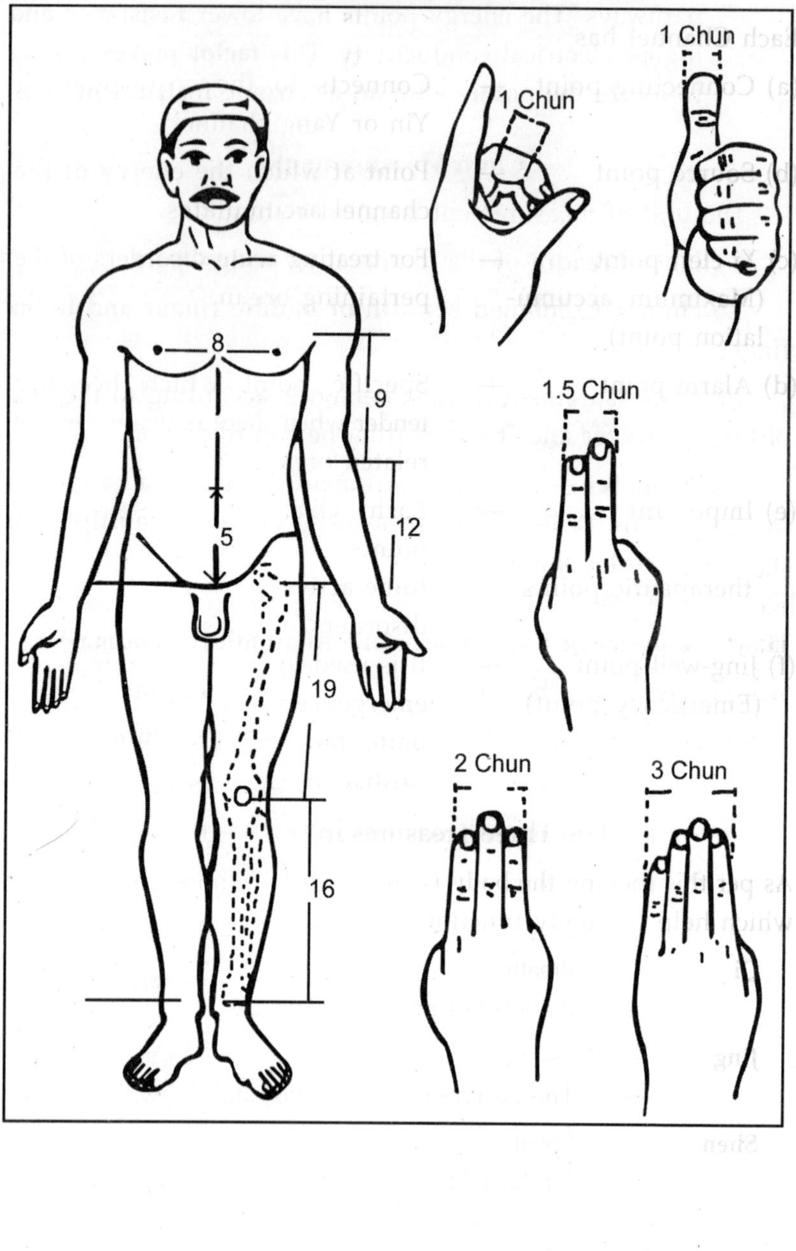

Points to be Noted of Each Channel

Each Channel has

(a) Connecting point	—	Connects to the corresponding Yin or Yang channel
(b) Source point	—	Point at which the energy of the channel accumulates.
(c) Xi cleft point (Maximum accumulation point)	—	For treating acute disorders of the pertaining organ.
(d) Alarm point	—	Specific point which becomes tender when there is disease of the related organ.
(e) Important therapeutic points	—	Each channel has important points to be activated to solve different disorders.
(f) Jing-well point (Emergency point)	—	It is used for treating acute emergencies like coma, severe pain, fainting, epileptic attack, cardiac arrest, shock, etc.

The Three Treasures in the Body

As per this therapy the body is endowed with three vital energies which help the body function. They are:

Qi	—	Breath
	—	It nourishes, protects and warms.
Jing	—	Essence
	—	This governs our constitution and ability to produce.
Shen	—	Spirit
	—	It is linked to heart. It helps in clear thinking.

The Vital Fluids

Blood — It is connected with Qi. It supplies nourishment throughout the body.

Jin — Water fluid. Moistens skin and hair.

Ye — Thick fluid. Lubricates joints, sense organ, brain and spinal cord. Affected in arthritic condition.

By activating the energy points these energies and fluids are stimulated and maintained, thus aiding the healthy functioning of body.

7

The Fourteen Channels

Location and Function

1.	Lung	—	Lu.
2.	Large intestine	—	L.I.
3.	Stomach	—	St.
4.	Spleen	—	Sp.
5.	Heart	—	H.
6.	Small intestine	—	S.I.
7.	Urinary bladder	—	U.B.
8.	Kidney	—	K.
9.	Pericardium	—	P.
10.	Triple Heater	—	T.H.
11.	Gall bladder	—	G.B.
12.	Liver	—	Li
13.	Governing vessel	—	Du
14.	Conception vessel	—	Ren

Functional Use of Meridians

EACH of the meridians listed in the therapy has multi-therapeutic function. They are connected to respective organs through internal channels.

The pressure points present in each channel act as mini transformers and when activated by applying pressure, help in treating various disorders, which may be pertaining to the organ connected, pertaining to the corresponding sense organ and tissue, local problems on the body lying along the pathway of the channel, or distal problems where the transfer of the energy to the distal point takes place through internal connections.

1. Lung Channel

Route — It is a Yin channel. **Organ time** - 3.00 am - 5.00 am

It starts from the upper part of the chest, 6 chun lateral to midline, at the interspace between 1st and 2nd rib. Then runs along the inner side of the arm along the outer margin till the wrist. From the wrist descends to the palm and ends at the base of the nail of the thumb, in the outer side.

Connection — Lung channel is connected to the large intestine channel.

The lungs are reponsible for absorbing Qi from the air and distributing it to all parts of the body. Lung also controls the part of the fluid metabolism which distributes the fluids to the skin.

Important — Lung **governs** skin and body hair.

— Lung **opens** to the nose.

— The **colour** of the skin becomes white on underfunctioning of lungs.

— The **emotion** is grief on underfunctioning.

— It is connected to **Element** : Metal, **Taste** : Pungent, **Odour** : Rank

Disharmony — Coughing, shortness of breath, white complexion, phlegm, skin problem, sadness and oppression.

It has eleven pressure points

The commonly used ones are — Lu 1, 5, 6, 7, 9 and 11.

Lu. 1 — At the interspace between 1st and 2nd rib, 6 chun lateral to the mid line.

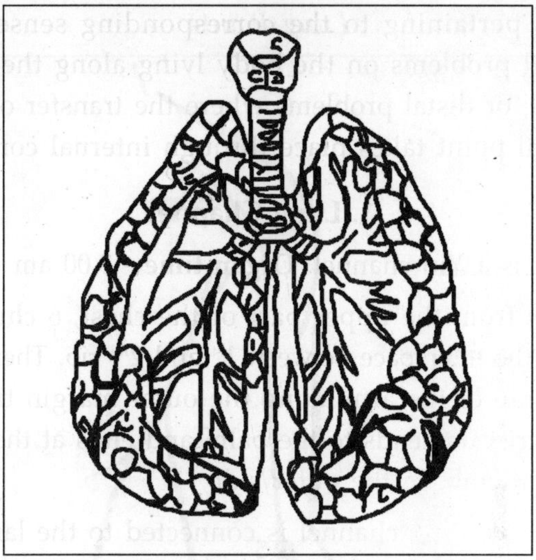

— Alarm point of the lung. It is tender on under functioning of the lungs.

Lu. 5 — At the level of the elbow crease, 1 chun inner to the edge of the elbow.

— Skin disease, pain or swelling of the elbow.

Lu. 6 — 5 chun distal to elbow crease on the Lu channel.

— Acute respiratory diseases.

Lu. 7 — 1.5 chun from the wrist crease along the Lu channel.

— An important distal point used for headache at the back and cervical spondylosis.

Lu. 9 — At the outer end of the wrist crease.

Influential point for vascular disorders.

Lu. 11 — 1 chun from outer corner of the nail of the thumb.

It is an emergency point.

Prick the point for hysterical attack. Fainting, epileptic attack, high fever, cardiac arrest, respiratory attack and other emergencies.

Lung Points

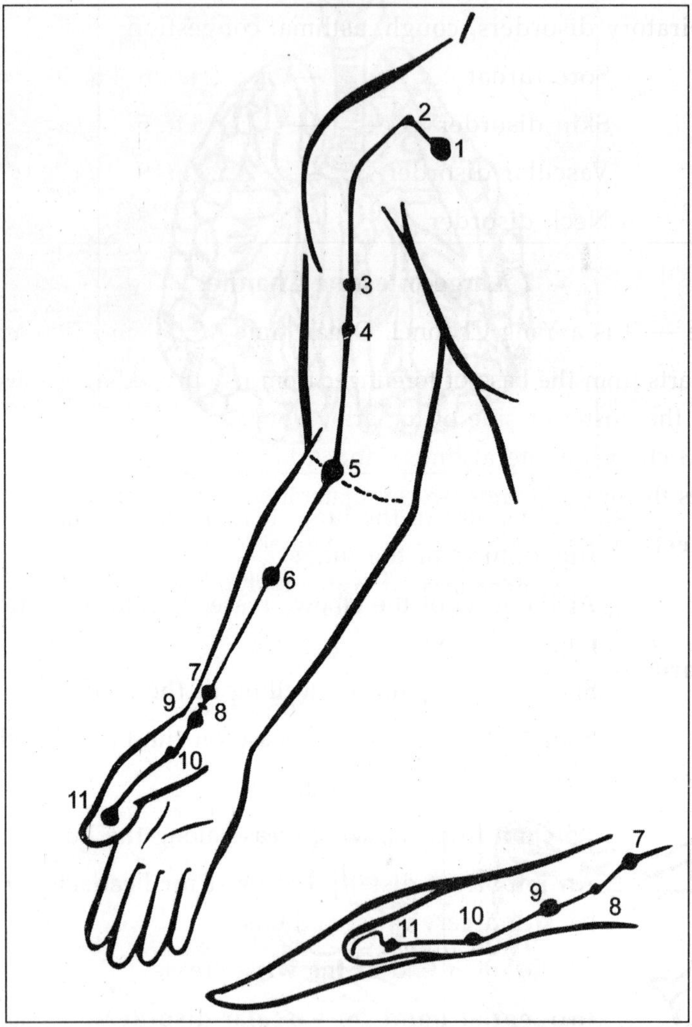

Source Point	— Lu. 9
Xi Cleft Point	— Lu. 6
Alarm Point	— Lu. 1
Connection Point	— Lu. 7

Five element points		
Lu.11	—	Wind point
Lu.10	—	Heat point
Lu.9	—	Earth point
Lu.8	—	**Dryness point**
Lu.5	—	Water point

Use of Points

Respiratory disorders, cough, asthma, congestion.

Sore throat	—	Lu. 6, Lu. 10
Skin disorder	—	Lu. 5
Vascular disorder	—	Lu. 9
Neck disorder	—	Lu. 7

2. Large Intestine Channel

Route — It is a Yang Channel. **Organ time** - 5.00 am - 7.00 am

Starts from the base of forefinger from its outer edge. It travels along the posterior side of the arm, along the shoulder over the neck 3 chun the lateral line of the Adam's apple, over the lips, crosses the lips and ends 0.5 chun lateral to the flair of the nostrils.

Connection — Large intestine channel is connected to lung. It takes care of water metabolism and excretion of waste.

Disharmony— Pain along the channel, frozen shoulder, pharyngitis, toothache, constipation, dry lips.

Large intestine

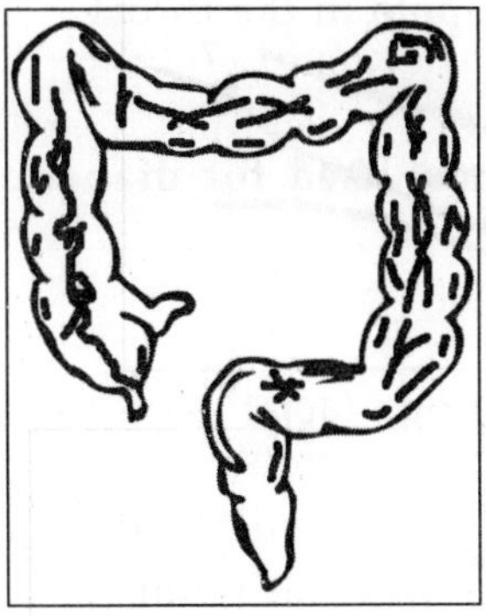

Large intestine Points

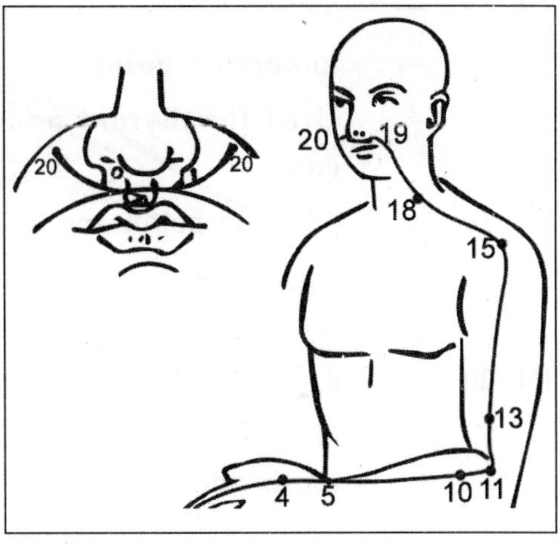

It has twenty pressure points

The commonly used ones are — L.I. 4, 10, 11, 15, 18, 19 and 20.

L.I. 4 — In the web angle between index finger and thumb, at the highest point of the muscles.

— **Best analgesic point.**

— For headache, front of the head and problems of sense organs on the face.

L.I. 10 — 2 chun below the crease of the elbow.

— Used for relieving pain. **It is a motor point.** For pain in forearm, tennis elbow, tremor or paralysis of the forearm.

L.I. 11 — At the outer end of the elbow crease, when the elbow is semi-flexed.

— **Best homoeostatic point of the body.** For high blood pressure, fevers, skin diseases.

L.I. 15 — 1.5 chun below the shoulder blade along the inner edge of the posterior arm.

— Disorders of the shoulder joint, frozen shoulder, paralysis of the arm.

L.I. 18 — 3 chun lateral to Adam's apple in the throat.

— **Endocrine point**

— **Used for thyroid problems, used for diabetic cure.**

L.I. 19 — 0.5 chun below the nose.

— Nasal block, nasal bleeding, facial paralysis, toothache.

L.I. 20 — 0.5 chun lateral to the nose flair.

— Nose block, nose bleeding, swollen face, toothache.

Source Point	—	L.I. 4
Connection Point	—	L.I.6
Xi Cleft Point	—	L.I. 7

Five element points		
L.I.1	**—**	**Dryness point**
L.I.2	—	Water point
L.I.4	—	Wind point
L.I.5	—	Heat point
L.I.11	—	Earth point

Use of Points		
Pain relief **(Best analgesic point)**	—	L.I. 4
Fever, high blood pressure. Skin disorders **(Best homoeostatic point)**	—	L.I. 11
Frozen shoulder	—	L.I. 15
Thyroid gland disorder	—	L.I. 18
Blocked nose, toothache, nasal discharge	—	L.I. 19, L.I. 20

3. Stomach Channel

Route — It is a Yang channel. **Organ time** - 7.00 am - 9.00 am

Starts its course below the eye. After running in a straight course till the jaw, it takes a U-turn outwards goes up till 0.5 chun lateral to anterior hairline. Then from the bottom of the U-turn the meridian continues downward along the neck. Near the collar-bone it goes laterally 4 chun to the midline till it reaches 1 chun below nipple line. There it turns inwards and runs 2 chun to the midline till the bottom of the abdomen.

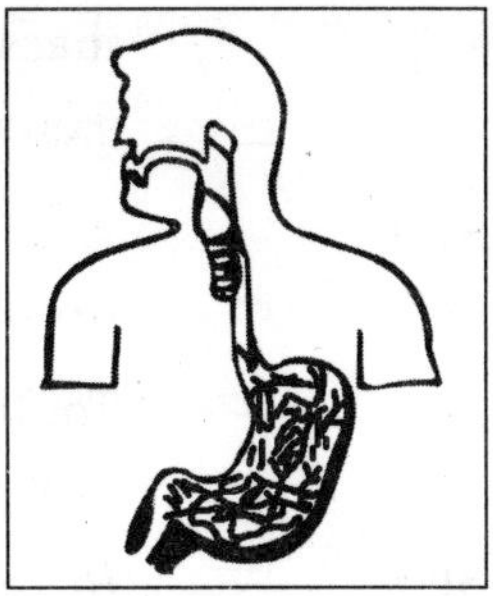

Then it runs along the outer side of the leg and ends at the base of the nail of the second toe.

Connection — Stomach channel is connected to spleen channel.

The stomach helps in digestion and transporta-tion of food and water.

Disharmony— Mental disturbance, deviation of eyes and mouth, feverish, pain and cramps on the outer side of the leg and dorsum of foot. Either overeating or food tasteless, gas, weakness in general.

It Has Forty-Five Pressure Points

The commonly used points are — St. 1 to St. 8, St. 18, 21, 25, 31, St. 32, 34, 38, 40, 41, 43 and 44.

St. 1 — Below the midpoint of the inner eyelid.

— Disorders of the eye and the eyelid.

St. 2 — 0.7 chun below St. 1.

— Eye disease, facial paralysis.

St. 3 — 1 chun below St. 2.

— Excessive salivation, speech difficulties, disorders of the upper teeth, mutism.

St. 5 — At the lowest point of the anterior border of the masseter muscle.

— Toothache, swelling of the cheek, facial paralysis.

St. 6 — At the prominent point of the muscle brought up on clenching the jaw. **A motor point.**

— Toothache, facial paralysis, spasm of the jaw muscle.

St. 7 — In the depression of the zygomatic arch.

— Toothache, deafness, vertigo, facial paralysis, sinusitis, headache.

St. 8 — 0.5 chun lateral to the anterior hairline.

Stomach Channel

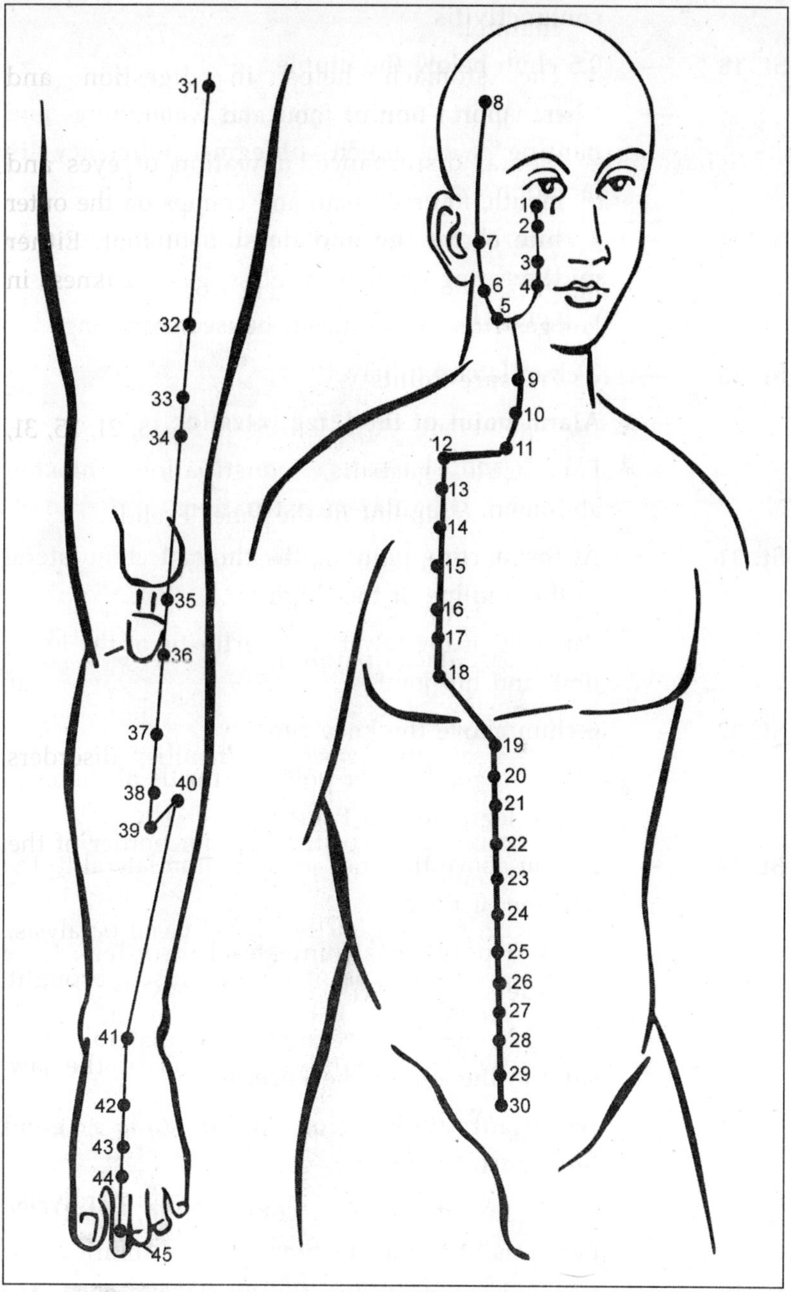

— Temporal headache, eye pain, sinusitis, conjunctivitis.

St. 18 — 0.5 chun below the nipple.

— Chest pain, angina pectoris, coughing and panting with much phlegm, deficiency in lactation.

St. 21 — 4 chun above the navel and 2 chun lateral to midline.

— For gastritis, peptic ulcer, nausea, vomiting.

St. 25 — 2 chun lateral to navel.

— **Alarm point of the large intestine.**

— For acute gastritis, constipation, bloated abdomen, irregular menstruation.

St. 31 — At the starting point of the thigh. 1 chun lateral to the midline of the thigh.

— Paralysis of the lower limb, arthritis of the lower limb and hip joint.

St. 32 — 6 chun above the knee cap.

— This is a good motor point. Arthritis of the knee severe leg pain and Paralysis.

St. 34 — 2 chun above the knee joint. 1 chun lateral to the midline of thigh.

— **Xi cleft point,** gastrointestinal disorders, knee disorders.

St. 36 — Found below the knee joint. 1 chun lateral (outer side) to the end of the kneecap.

— **Important tonification point and a good homoeostatic point.**

— Used for diarrhoea, constipation, gastritis, paralysis of the lower limb, general tonification.

St. 37 — 2 chun from St. 36.

— **Used for acute appendicitis**, large intestine disorders.

St. 38 — 5 chun below St. 36

Frozen shoulder. By manipulating this point there can be dramatic improvement in frozen shoulder.

St. 40 — 1 chun lateral to St. 38

— **It is the connecting point to spleen, an important point.**

— Cough, excessive sputum, epilepsy.

St. 41 — On the ankle crease.

— Varicose vein, chronic ulcers in the ankle area, foot drop.

St. 43 — 2 chun below base of the 2nd and 3rd toes.

— **A good analgesic (pain remover) point.** The point is effective for headaches, swollen face, leg pain.

St. 44 — Found between the web of 2nd and 3rd toes. 0.5 chun above the web.

— **Best analgesic point of the lower limb, distal point too** for toothache, headache, abdominal pain, etc.

Source Point	—	St. 42
Connection Point	—	St. 40
Xi Cleft Point	—	St. 34

Five element points

St.45	—	Dryness point
St.44	—	Water point
St.43	—	Wind point
St.40	—	Heat point
St.36	—	**Earth point**

Use of Points

Paralysis of the face, deviation of eyes and mouth	—	St. 1 to 7
Toothache	—	St. 4, 5, 6, 7, 44
Sinusitis and temporal headache	—	St. 7, 8, 44

Gastric problem	—	St. 21, 25
Diarrhoea, constipation, indisposition	—	St. 34, 36
General tonification	—	St. 36
(A Good tonification and homoeostatic point)		
Pain in knees	—	St. 35, 36
Leg pain	—	St. 32
Facial oedema, headache	—	St. 44
(Best analgesic point of the lower limb)		

4. Spleen Channel

Route — It is a Yin channel. **Organ time** - 9.00 am - 11.00 am

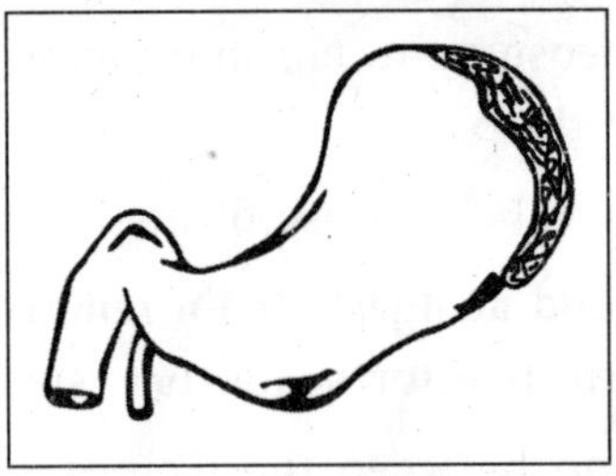

It starts from the inner side of the big toe. Then it travels along the inner side of the leg, climbs up the abdomen, goes further to the chest, takes a turn above the nipples and ends below the armpit.

Connection — The spleen channel is connected to stomach channel. Spleen helps in digestion and transportation of food. It aids in production of blood and Qi. It controls water metabolism.

Importance — Spleen governs the soft tissues, muscle tendons, inside of the mouth, lining of the organs, holding the viscera (internal organs) in place, fat and the four limbs.

Spleen **opens** to the mouth.

The **colour** of lips becomes yellow on under-functioning. The **emotion** is obsession and unproductive thoughts. It is connected to **Element**: Earth, **Taste**: Sweetness. **Odour:** Fragrant.

Spleen influences weight problem. Determines the form of body and distribution of flesh. Obesity is associated with it.

Spleen is responsible for holding abdominal organs in correct position. Many instances of prolapse are due to weakened spleen.

Spleen Channel

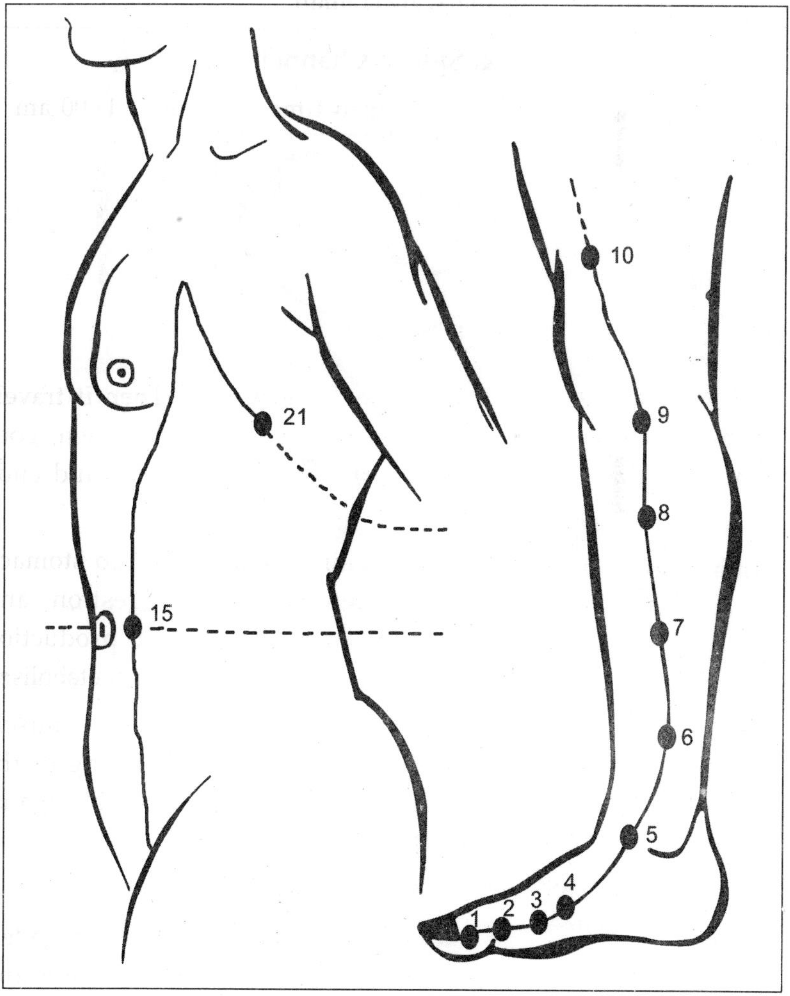

Spleen Channel

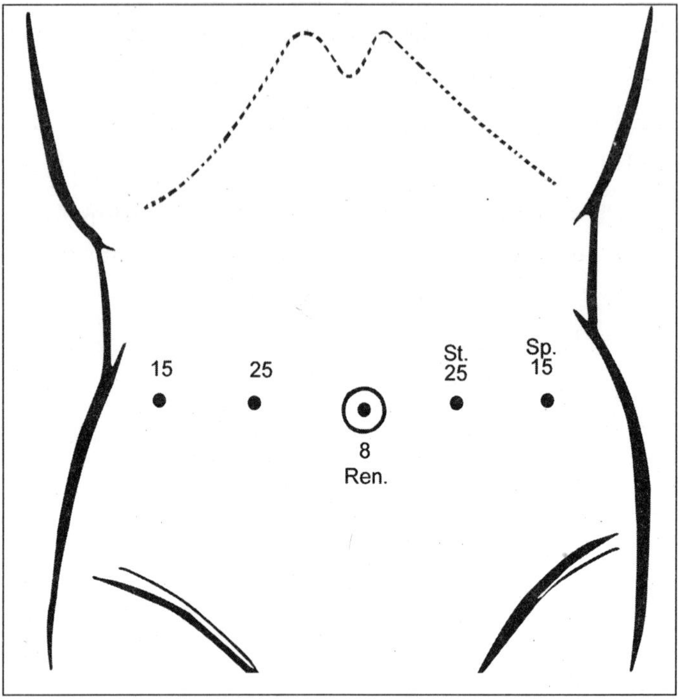

It prevents leakage of blood from blood vessel. Haemorrhage is linked to spleen.

As spleen is responsible for transporting nourishment, a weak spleen leads to general lassitude, weakness and pale complexion.

Disharmony — Fatigue, tendency to lie down and rest, weak flesh, eruption of gas from stomach, digestive problems, nausea, vomiting, prolapse, thoughts going round and round, pain at the root of the tongue.

It has 21 Pressure points

The commonly used ones are Sp. 4, 6, 9, 10, 15.

Sp. 4 — On the foot in the depression below 1st metacarpal bone.

— It is the **connecting point** to stomach.

— Very acute diarrhoea, pain in the intestine, ulcers.

Sp. 6 — 3 chun above the ankle bone on the inner side.

— 3 Yin channels (kidney, liver, spleen) meet here.

— One of the **best tonification points.** All gastro-intestinal, genito-urinary disorders, skin disorders, mouth disorders are improved by stimulating this point.

Sp. 9 — 2 chun below the knee joint in the depression after the joint along the inner side.

— A good point to check oedema or **swelling in the body.**

Sp. 10 — 2 chun above the knee joint towards the inner side of the thigh. If the palm is rested on the knee joint of the patient, the place where the tip of the thumb falls, lies this point.

— For all kinds of allergies, skin diseases and menstrual problems.

Sp. 15 — 4 chun lateral to the navel.

— **Best point for gas related problems.**

Sp. 21 — In the space between 6th and 7th ribs. Below the arm-pit along the side of the chest.

— **It is a major connection point.**

— It relieves chest pain. Harmonises right and left, upper and lower, inside and outside of body.

Source Point	—	Sp. 3
Xi Cleft Point	—	Sp. 8
Connection Point	—	Sp. 4 and Sp. 21

Five element points		
Sp.1	—	Wind point
Sp.2	—	Heat point
Sp.3	**—**	**Earth point**
Sp.5	—	Dryness point
Sp.9	—	Water point

Use of Points		
Acute diarrhoea	—	Sp. 4
For tonification of metabolic organs	—	Sp. 6
(a good tonification point)		
Menstrual problems	—	Sp. 6, Sp. 10
Gastric problems	—	Sp. 6 to Sp. 10
Oedema —		Sp. 9
(Effective point for swelling)		
Skin disorder, allergies, immune disorders	—	Sp. 6, Sp. 10
(a good point for allergy problems)		
Ulcers in mouth, vomiting, belching	—	Sp. 6, 15, 21

5. Heart Channel

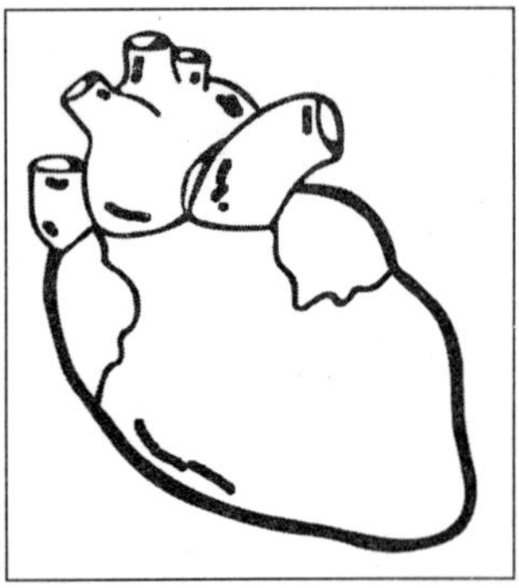

Route - It is a Yin channel.
Organ time - 11.00 am - 1.00 pm

It originates from the chest close to the armpit, then runs along the medial aspect of the arm in the inner side and over the palm and ends near the base of the little finger.

Heart controls the blood vessel and the circulation of the blood.

Heart also stores the spirit hence it is associated with the mental processes and working of the brain. In this therapy as there is no separate channel to control brain functions, it is the heart and pericardium channel which controls the working of brain and mental activity.

Connection — Heart is connected to small intestine channel.

Importance — Heart **governs** blood vessels and brain (nervous system). Heart **opens** to tongue.

The **colour** of mouth and tongue turns red when heart malfunctions.

It is connected to **Element**: Fire, **Emotion:** Laughter, **Taste**: bitterness, **Odour:** burning.

Disharmony — Pain along the inner aspect of the arm, night sweating, dryness of throat, emotional distress, dizziness, palpitation, lack of vitality, insomnia, restlessness.

It has 9 acupressure points.

The commonly used ones are H. 3, 5, 6, 7, 8, 9

H. 3 — On the elbow crease. One to the inner side.

— Disorder of the elbow, numbness of the forearm, chest pain, angina pectoris.

H. 5 — 1 chun from H.7 - (**connection point**)

— Hoarseness of voice, stammering (heart is connected to tongue).

H. 6 — 0.5 chun from H. 7

— **The Xi cleft point of the channel.**

— Treats acute heart diseases — Angina pectoris, palpitation, severe depression, maniacal behaviour (as heart is connected to brain), suddenly dumb, night sweats.

H. 7 — Along the side of the little finger, on the wrist crease over the cubital artery.

— **Important tranquilliser point.**

— Rhythm disorders of the heart, anxiety, mental disorders, insomnia, shortness of breath, palpitation, cardiac oedema, cold sweat.

H. 8 — On the palm. Between the tips of ring finger and little finger on tightly clenching the fist.

— Disorders of the palm. Arthritis of the finger joint.

H.9 — 0.1 chun to the inner corner of the nail of the little finger.

— **It is an emergency point.**

Heart Channel

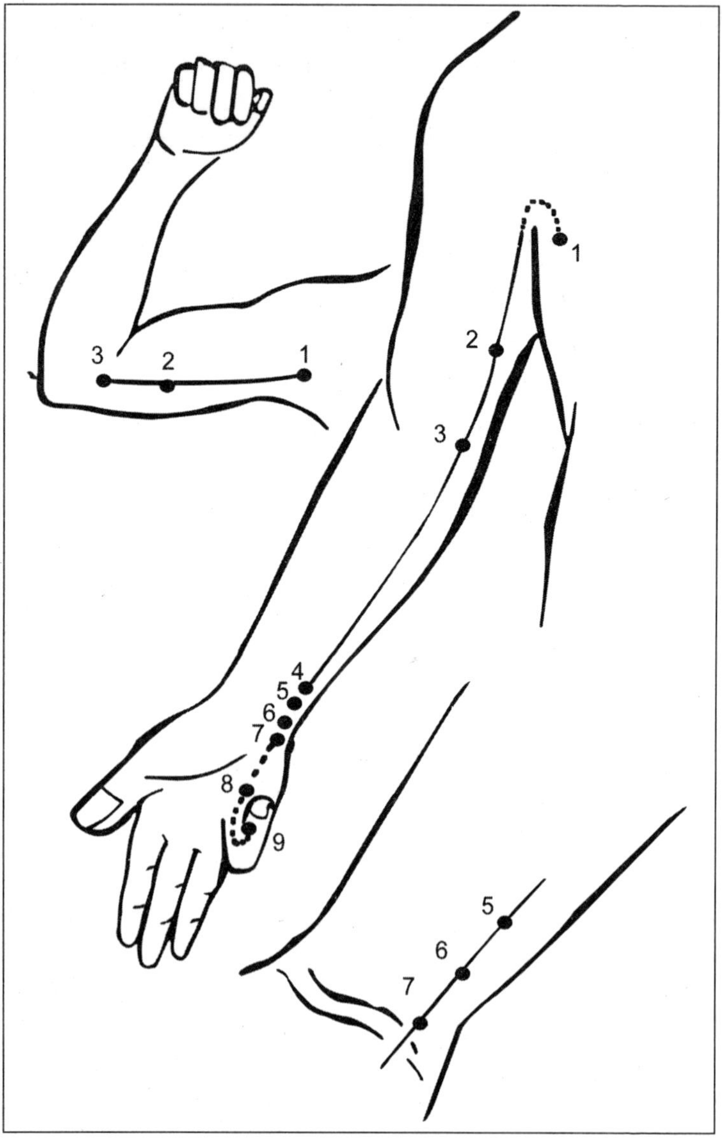

— Palpitation, pain in the chest, dry throat, lack of energy and other acute emergencies.

Source Point	— H. 7
Xi Cleft Point	— H. 6
Connection Point	— H. 5

Five element points		
H.9	—	Wind point
H.8	—	**Heat point**
H.7	—	Earth point
H.4	—	Dryness point
H.3	—	Water point

Use of Points		
Heart disease, angina pectoris, palpitation, missing rhythm.	—	H. 4, H. 5, H. 7
Mental disorders **(Heart is connected to brain)**	—	H. 6, H. 7
Insomnia **(A good tranquilliser point)**	—	H. 7
Hoarseness of voice **(Heart is connected to tongue)**	—	H. 5

6. Small Intestine Channel

Route — It is a Yang channel. **Organ time** - 1.00 pm -3.00 pm

It starts from the outer end of the little finger, then runs along the rim of the outer side of the arm, zigzags over the shoulder, runs over the neck and then travels to the cheek and ends near the ear.

Small intestine separates the essence and waste from the food, the essence with the help of spleen is distributed in the body and waste is passed to the large intestine.

Connection — S.I. is connected to heart.

Disharmony— Pain along the channel in the arms, temporal headache, deafness or pain around ears, swelling of the cheek, lower abdominal pain.

Small Intestine Channel

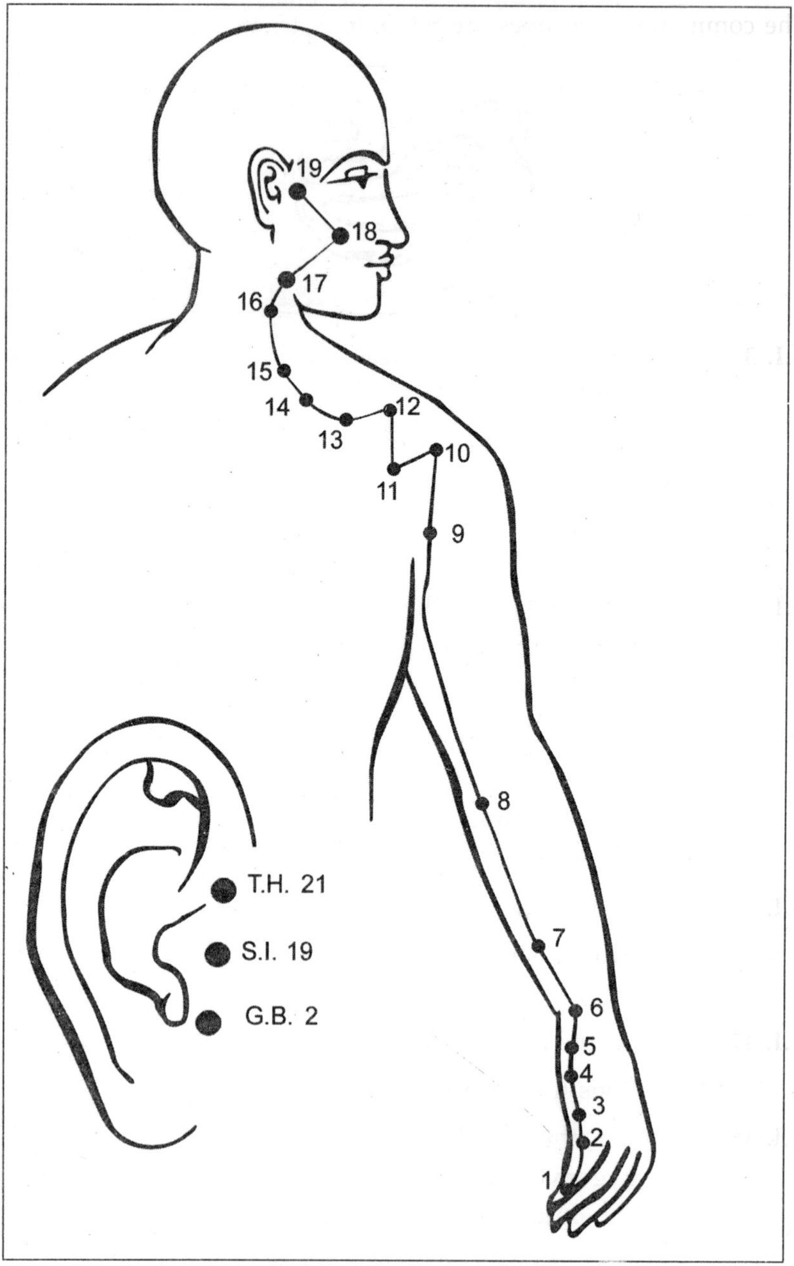

It has 19 Acupressure points

The commonly used ones are S.I. 3, 6, 9, 17, 18, 19

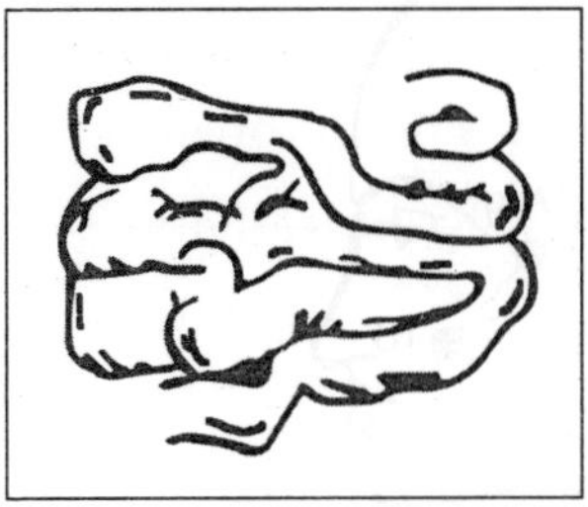

S.I. 3 — At the end of the crease of the palm on clenching the fist.

— Acute stiffness of neck, spasm and pain in the arm, occipital headache, night sweats, epilepsy, deafness.

(It is the confluence point of Du channel.)

S.I. 6 — On the back of the wrist along the little finger in the depression behind the wrist bone.

— **Xi cleft point.**

— Pain in the wrist, pain in the arms, cervical spondylosis, stiff neck is dramatically relieved by strong stimulation of this point. Failing vision in elderly.

S.I. 9 — 1 chun above the crease of the armpit.

— Frozen shoulder, pain or paralysis of the upper limb.

S.I. 17 — At the angle of the jaw.

— Tonsillitis, sore throat.

S.I. 18 — On the cheek, below the prominence of the zygomatic bone, on the vertical line drawn from the outer corner of the eye.

— **Best regional analgesic (pain remover) joint.**

— Used to treat effectively toothache, facial paralysis, eyes blinking.

S.I. 19 — Close to the ears in the depression when the mouth is slightly open.

— Ear disorders (deafness), vertigo.

Source Point	—	S.I. 4
Xi Cleft Point	—	S.I. 6
Connection Point	—	S.I. 7

Five element points		
S.I.1	—	Dryness point
S.I.2	—	Water point
S.I.3	—	Wind point
S.I.5	**—**	**Heat point**
S.I.8	—	Earth point

Use of Points		
Stiff neck, cervical spondylosis	—	S.I. 6, S.I. 3
Failing vision in elderly	—	S.I. 6
Shoulder pain	—	S.I. 9
Tonsillitis, sore throat	—	S.I. 17
Toothache	—	S.I. 18
(a good analgesic point)		
Ear disorder (deafness)	—	S.I. 19

7. Urinary Bladder Channel

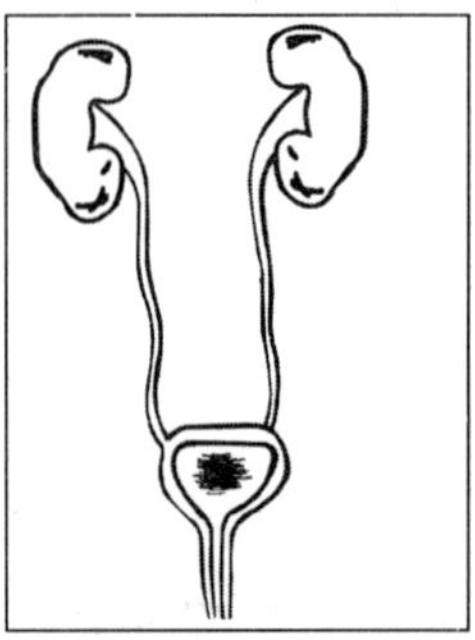

Route - It is a Yang channel.
Organ time - 3.00pm - 5.00pm

The channel begins close to the inner corner of the eye near the nose, from there it travels up over the head and descends to the nape of the neck. There it divides into two branches.

One branch which is more frequently used in therapy travels 1.5 chun lateral to the spinal column till it reaches the 4th sacral vertebra at the lower back. There it takes an oblique route, goes up to the 1st

Urinary Bladder Channel

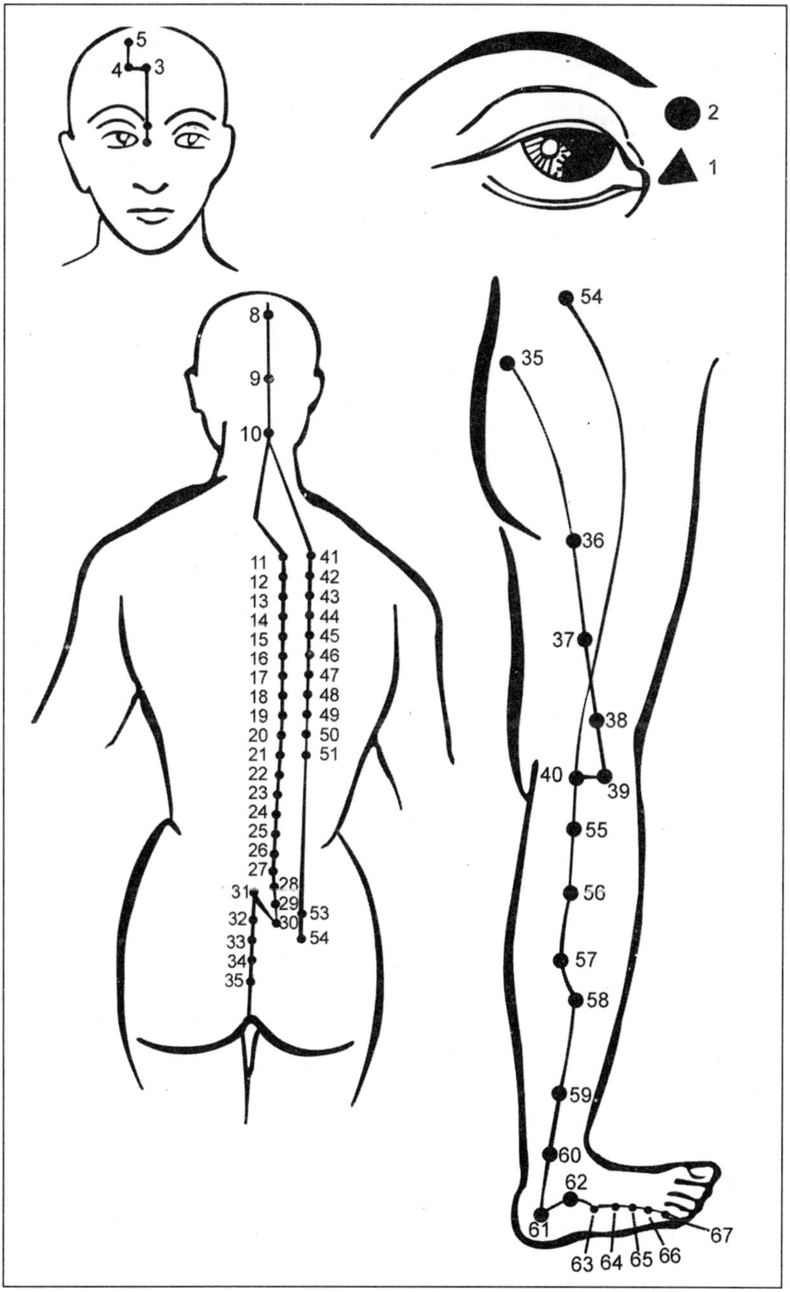

sacral vertebra and then descends close to the spinal cord till coccyx and further goes along the back of the lower limb.

The other branch travels 3 chun lateral to the spinal cord straight down along the lower back, over to the buttocks then to the lower limb along the back. Behind the knee joint it meets the first branch. From here both the branches become one.

They then travel downwards over the calf muscle on to the foot, circles around the ankle and ends in the lateral corner of the last toe.

Urinary bladder collects fluid from different parts of the body and expels as urine. It is responsible for water balance.

Disharmony — Pain in the back along the spinal column, sciatica, vertical and occipital headache.

It has 67 Acupressure points.

It is a therapeutically important channel having **12 alarm points** treating variety of disorders.

The important ones are —

Face — U.B. 1 and 2.

Neck — U.B. 10.

Trunk — U.B. 11, 13, 14, 15, 17, 18, 19, 20, 21, 22, 23, 24, 25, 27, 28 and 32.

Lower limb — U.B. 36, 40, 57, 58, 60, 62 and 67.

U.B. 1 — 0.1 chun to the inner corner of the eye.
— Eye disorders.

U.B. 2 — In the depression at the inner end of the eyebrow.
— Eye disorders, sinusitis, frontal headache.

U.B. 10 — 1.3 chun lateral to the spinal column, between the 1st and 2nd vertebrae of the neck.
— Stiff neck, cervical spondylosis, occipital headache.

U.B. 11 — 1.5 chun lateral to the spinal column along the lower border of the 1st thoracic vertebra.

— **Influential point for the bone and cartilage.**

— Used for all joint, bone and cartilage disorders.

U.B. 13 — 1.5 chun lateral to the spinal column along the lower border of third thoracic vertebra.

— **Back alarm point of the lungs.**

— Lung disorders, skin disorders (as skin is connected to the lungs).

U.B. 14 — 1.5 chun lateral to the spinal column along the lower border of 4th thoracic Vertebra

— **Back alarm point of pericardium**

— Heart disease, Brain disorders.

U.B. 15 — 1.5 chun to spinal column along the lower border of 5th thoracic vertebra.

— **Back alarm point of the heart.**

— Heart diseases. Brain disorders, epilepsy, hysteria, insomnia.

U.B. 17 — 1.5 chun to spinal column along the lower border of 7th thoracic vertebra.

— **Back alarm point of the diaphragm.**

— **Influential point for blood and blood related disorders. Anaemia, leukaemia, hiccough.**

U.B. 18 — 1.5 chun to the spinal column along the lower border of the 9th thoracic vertebra.

— **Back alarm point of the liver.**

— Liver disease, eye disorders, muscle and tendon disorders. (Since liver is connected to the sense organ eye and to the tissue muscle and tendon.)

Note: S.C — Spinal Column

U.B. 19 — 1.5 chun to the spinal column along the lower border of the 10th thoracic vertebra.

— **Back alarm point of the gall bladder.**

— Gall bladder disorders.

U.B. 20 — 1.5 chun to the spinal column along the lower border of the 11th thoracic vertebra.

— **Back alarm point of the spleen.**

— Spleen disorders. Treats allergies. Gastrointestinal problems, oedema, soft tissue disorders (spleen is connected to soft tissue like inside of the mouth, stomach lining, nose lining, etc.).

U.B. 21 — 1.5 chun to the spinal column along the lower border of the 12th thoracic vertebra.

— **Back alarm point of the stomach.**

— Stomach disorders.

U.B. 22 — 1.5 chun to the spinal column along the lower border of the 1st lumbar vertebra.

— **Back alarm point of the Triple heater, which controls the three body cavities.**

— Abdominal distension, flatulence, loss of appetite, incontinence of urine.

U.B. 23 — 1.5 chun to the spinal column along the lower border of the 2nd lumbar vertebra.

— **Back alarm point of the kidney.**

— Genito-urinary disorders, ear disease, bone disorders, baldness (kidney is connected to the sense organ ear and to the tissue bone and head hair).

U.B. 25 — 1.5 chun to the spinal column along the lower border of the 4th lumbar vertebra.

— **Back alarm point of large intestine.**

— Diarrhoea, constipation, low backache.

U.B. 27 — 1.5 chun to the spinal column along the lower border of first sacral vertebra.

— **Back alarm point of small intestine.**

— Diarrhoea, blood in stools, low backache.

U.B. 28 — 1.5 chun to the spinal column along the lower border of the second sacral vertebra.

— **Back alarm point of urinary bladder.**

— Genito-urinary disorders.

U.B. 32 — On the second sacral vertebra.

— Genital diseases of both the sexes, haemorrhoids.

U.B. 54 — 3 chun to the 4th sacral vertebra.

— Hip disorders, sciatica, bleeding haemorrhoids.

U.B. 36 — In the middle of the gluteal fold.

— Sciatica, low backache.

U.B. 40 — At the midpoint in the crease behind the knee-cap.

— **One of the 6 important distal points.**

— Sciatica, paralysis of the lower limb, disorders of the knee joint, skin diseases.

U.B. 57 — 8 chun to U.B. 40.

— Cramps in the calf muscle, pain in the foot, paralysis of the lower limb.

U.B. 58 — 1 chun inferior and lateral to U.B. 57.

— Weakness of the legs, an irritable bladder, opthalmoplegia (**improves the eyesight).**

U.B. 60 — In the curve of the heel bone behind ankle.

— Painful ankle conditions, foot swollen, sciatica, paralysis of the lower limbs.

U.B. 62 — 0.5 chun to the lower border of the ankle at the back.

— **Important sedative point in the body.** Helps in epilepsy, mental illnesses, drug addictions, insomnia, tension headache.

U.B. 67 — 0.1 chun lateral to the end of the little toe nail.

— Helps in difficult labour but abortion may be caused in early months of pregnancy. Difficulty in urination.

Source Point	—	U.B. 64
Connection Point	—	U.B. 58

Five element points		
U.B.67	—	Dryness point
U.B.66	**—**	**Water point**
U.B.64	—	Wind point
U.B.60	—	Heat point
U.B.40	—	Earth point

Use of Points

U.B. channel treats variety of diseases. Located 1.5 chun to either side of spine, it has twelve alarm points of different important organs as shown in alarm points diagram.

It has Two Influential Points

1. Bone and cartilage	—U.B. 11
2. Blood	—U.B. 17
It has Twelve Alarm Points	—U.B. 13 to 28
The channel then runs back of the leg treating the leg troubles, Pain in the leg, calf muscles.	—U.B. 40 to U.B. 57
Mental disorders, insomnia, drug addictions	—U.B. 62

(A good sedative point)

8. Kidney Channel

Route — It is a Yin channel. **Organ time** - 5.00 pm - 7.00 pm

It begins at the sole of the foot, travels up along the inner side of the ankle to the leg, traverses the leg along the inner side, climbs up the abdomen, travelling close to the midline it ends in the upper part of the chest.

Kidneys are the roots of life. They store Jing, the essence of the life, which is responsible for growth, development and reproductive functions. The strength of kidney determines the strength of the constitution. Kidney has both Yin and Yang. The Yin is the water element and the Yang is fire. Any disorder, sufficiently chronic, will involve kidney. Acupuncture points for kidney Yang is at the level of waist on the spine. It increases

Kidney Channel

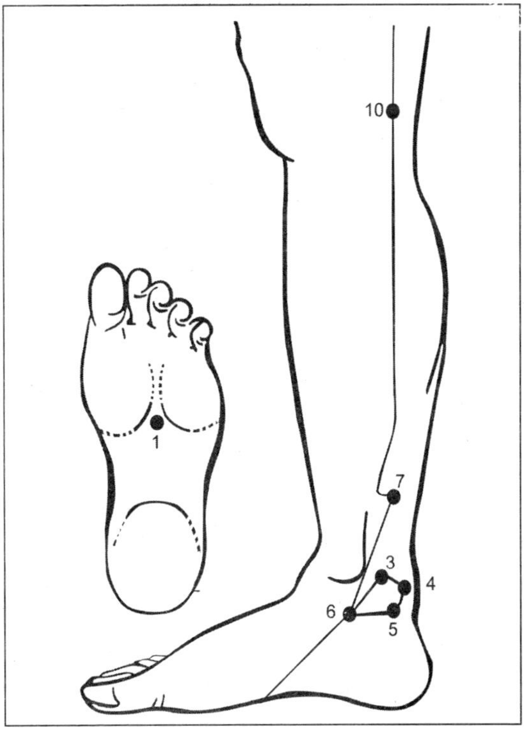

the basic energy level and tonifies. Kidney influences the water metabolism and control of body fluids.

Connection — Kidney is connected to urinary bladder channel.

Importance — Kidney **governs** bone and cartilage, teeth and hair on the head.

Kidney **opens** to the ears.

The **colour** of the medial side of forearm becomes black. It is connected to the **Element:** water, **Emotion:** fear, **Colour:** black, **Odour:** rotten smell, **Sound:** groaning.

Disharmony — Lack of energy, low backache, dark circles under eyes, dizziness, tinnitus (constant ringing in ears), feverish sensation of the soles, weakness of lower limbs, irregular menstruation, impotence.

It has 27 acupressure points

The commonly used ones are K 1, 3, 5, 6, 7, 10, 27.

K 1 — In the sole of the foot. In a straight line below the 2nd and 3rd toe in the depression below.

— **It is very effective point used for various emergencies.**

— For fainting, coma, shock, hysteria, epileptic attack, infantile convulsions and hypertension.

K 3 — 0.5 chun lateral and 0.5 chun above the lower border of the inner ankle. **It is the source point.**

— Genito-urinary disorders, impotence, irregular menstruation, prolapse of the uterus, low backache, frequent asthmatic attacks.

K 4 — 0.5 chun inferior to K. 3 and along the outer end of the leg.

	—	**It is the connection point** to U.B. channel.
	—	Blurred vision, myopia, irregular period, menstrual distress, fear and unhappiness.
K 5	—	1 chun below K. 3. **It is the XI cleft point.** Renal colic, asthmatic attacks, prone to fear and unhappiness.
K 6	—	1 chun below the lower end of the ankle bone.
	—	Genito-urinary disorders (impotence, irregular menstruation), heel swollen and painful.
K 7	—	2 chun above K 3 close to the ankle.
	—	Excessive sweating, cold feet, bronchial asthma.
K 10	—	At the inner end of the knee crease on a straight line to K. 3.
	—	Knee disorders, impotence, urine dark yellow, vaginal discharge, baldness.
K 27	—	In the depression in the lower border of collar bone and 1st rib, 2 chun lateral to midline or Ren channel. The last point of the channel. **The Yin energy then flows to pericardium 1.**

Source Point	—	K. 3
Xi Cleft Point	—	K. 5
Connection Point	—	K. 4

Five element points		
K.1	—	Wind point
K.2	—	Heat point
K.3	—	Earth point
K.7	—	Dryness point
K.10	**—**	**Water point**

Use of Points

Kidney channel exercises its influence on urinary and genital organs.

Acute emergencies like fainting, coma, cardiac arrest, convulsion, high blood pressure	—	K. 1, K. 3

Urinary disorder, retention of urine, incontinence in urination, nocturnal emission, renal colic	—	K. 3, K. 5
Low backache, menstrual problems	—	K. 3, K. 5, K. 7
Asthma, congestion, sore throat	—	K. 3, K. 7
Oedema of the ankle	—	K. 6
Baldness, loss of hair, grey hair	—	K. 10

The kidney and the urinary bladder are connected to the bone, cartilage, to the head hair and to the sense organ ear.

9. Pericardium Channel

Route — It is a Yin channel. **Organ time** - 7.00 pm - 9.00 pm

It starts 1 chun lateral to the nipple in the chest travels along the inside of the arm between the lung channel and the heart channel and ends at the tip of the middle finger.

Pericardium is the lining of the heart. It is important in this therapy as, an energy channel is attached to this. Its functions are almost the same as heart. It regulates the working of blood and circulation. It is attached to brain and nervous system. It influences the working of mental processes.

Connection — It is connected to triple heater.

Disharmony — Poor sleep or insomnia, lack of energy, emotional distress, heavy headedness, palpitation.

It has 9 acupressure points

The commonly used ones are P. 3, 4, 5, 6, 7, 8

P. 3 — In the centre of the elbow crease.

— Angina pectoris, anxiety, dry mouth, pain at the elbow.

P. 4 — **It is a xi cleft point.** 5 chun from the wrist crease.

— It is used to treat acute heart and brain disorders. Angina pectoris, myocarditis, rhythm disorders,

Pericardium Channel

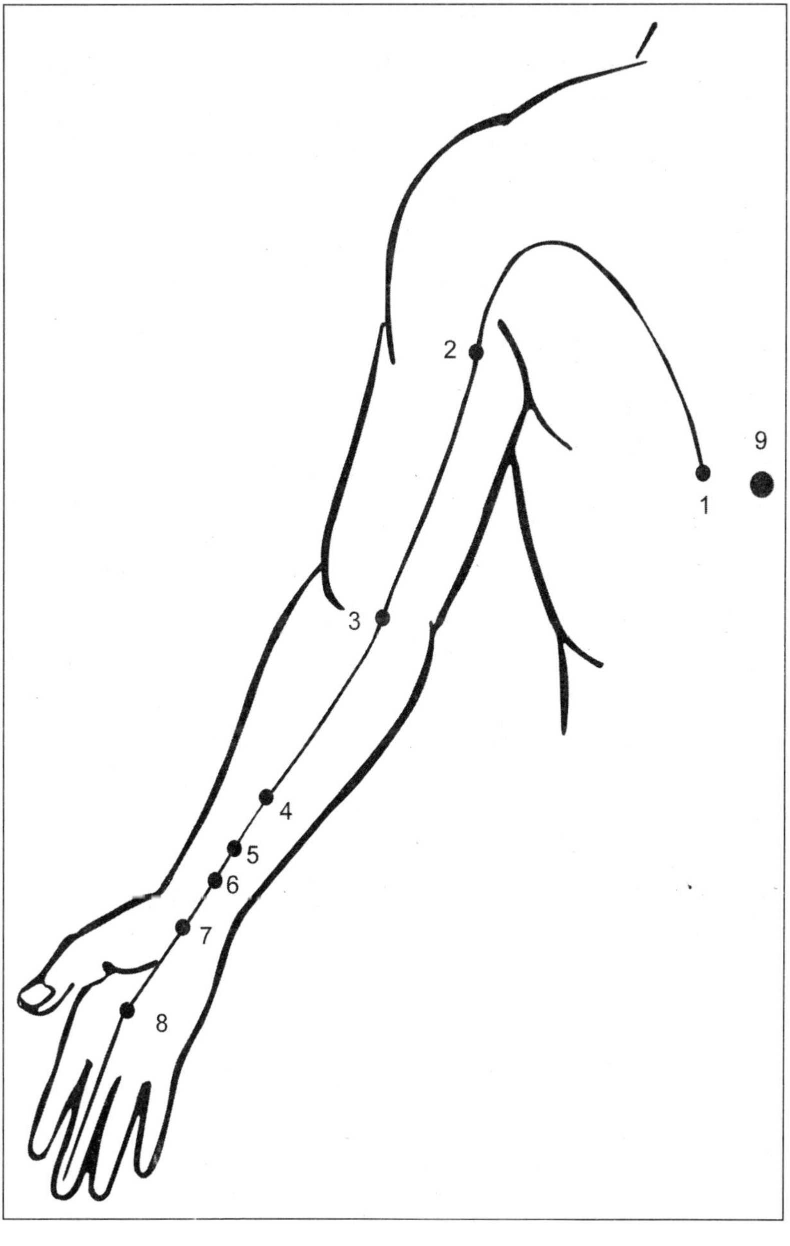

acute depression, hysteria, poor memory, lack of energy.

P. 6 — **An important distal point.** 2 chun from the wrist crease.

— **It is a connecting point to triple heater.** Hence apart from heart and brain disorders it is also used to treat chest and upper abdominal disorders.

Heart disease — Angina pectoris, palpitation.

Brain disease — Mental disorders, anxiety, insomnia, epilepsy.

Abdominal disorders — Pain in the chest, nausea, vomiting, peptic ulcer.

P. 7 — At the midpoint of the wrist crease.

— **It is a source point.** Disorders of the wrist joint.

P. 8 — On the palm. Between the tips of the middle finger and index finger when the fist is closed.

— Disorders of the palm, arthritis of the finger joints, excessive sweating of the palm.

Source Point	—	P. 7
Connection Point	—	P. 6
Xi Cleft Point	—	P. 4

Five element points		
P.9	—	Wind point
P.8	**—**	**Heat point**
P.7	—	Earth point
P.5	—	Dryness point
P.3	—	Water point

Use of Points

Heart disease, angina pectoris, palpitation, anxiety, cardiac rhythm disorders.	—	P. 3, P. 4, P. 6
Acute depression, mental disorders. **(Xi cleft point of pericardium)**	—	P. 4
Nausea, vomiting, gastritis, peptic ulcer	—	P. 6
Pain in the wrist joint	—	P. 7
Excessive sweating	—	P. 8

10. Triple Heater Channel (Sanjiao Channel)

Route — It is a Yang channel. **Organ time** - 9.00 pm - 11.00 pm

Starting from the lateral end of the ring finger it traverses the arm from outside, between the small intestine channel and the large intestine channel. From the shoulder it travels to the neck, circles the outer side of the ear, moves to the cheek and ends at the side of the eyebrow.

Triple Heater Channel

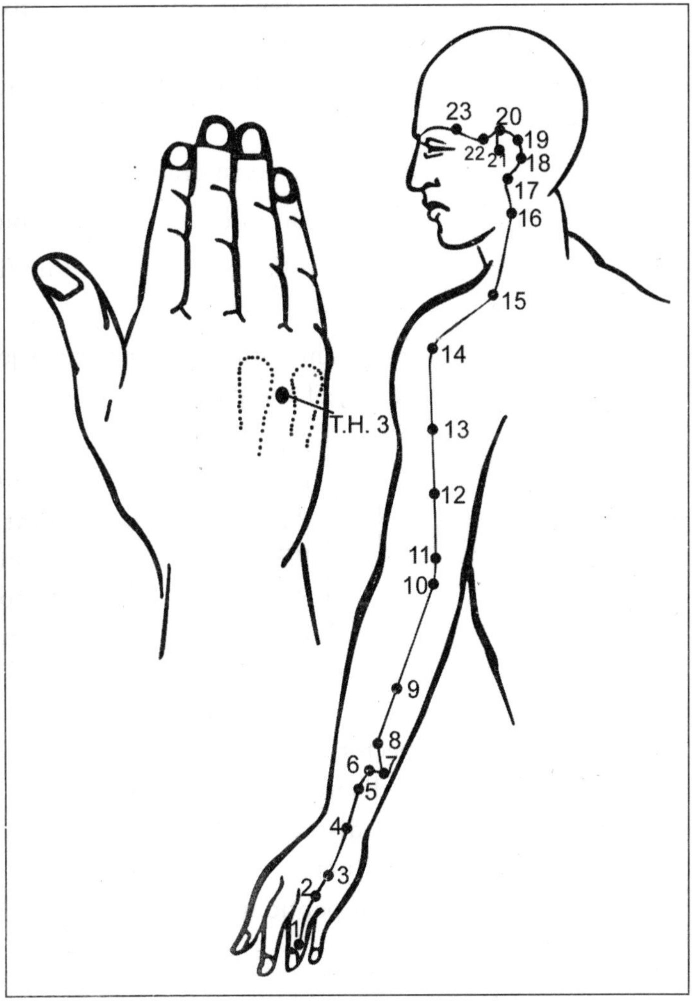

It harmonises the functions of all organs found in the body. It operates at three levels.

Upper heater — Chest, neck, head, heart and lungs.

Middle heater — Stomach and spleen.

Lower heater — Intestine, bladder and kidney.

It ensures the movement of Qi and fluids throughout the body.

Connection — T.H. is connected to pericardium.

Disharmony — Pain along the channel, eye-ear disorder, swelling in the body, coldness.

It has 23 accupressure points.

The commonly used ones are T.H. 3, 5, 6, 8, 14, 17, 20, 21 and 23.

T.H. 3 — On the dorsal side of the palm, between the heads of the 4th and 5th metacarpal bones.

— Ear disorders, deafness, ringing in the ears, pain in the arm.

T.H. 5 — 2 chun above the middle of the wrist crease on the dorsal side.

— **It is connection point to pericardium channel.**

— Headache along the forehead, acute pain in the arm, stiff neck, ear disorders.

T.H. 8 — 4 chun above the wrist crease.

— Effective in treating pain due to herpes, throat pain. Used for acupuncture anaesthesia for thoracic surgery.

T.H. 14 — When the arm is kept in the horizontal position, in the depression of the deltoid muscle, just below the shoulder.

— Frozen shoulder, pain in the arm, paralysis of the arm.

T.H. 17 — In the depression behind the ear lobe.

— Ear disorders, mumps, facial paralysis.

T.H. 20 — At the apex of the ear when the ear is folded.

— **It is an endocrine point.** Endocrine disorders like **Diabetes,** dwarfism, difficulty in chewing, gums swollen.

T.H. 21 — In front of the ear in the depression above the jaw bone, located more easily when the jaw is open.

— Ear disorders, toothache.

T.H. 23 — In the depression at the end of the eyebrow.

— Eye disease, temporal headache.

Source Point	—	T.H. 4
Connection Point	—	T.H. 5
Xi Cleft Point	—	T.H. 7

Five element points		
T.H.1	—	Dryness point
T.H.2	—	Water point
T.H.3	—	Wind point
T.H.5	**—**	**Heat point**
T.H.10	—	Earth point

Use of Points

It regulates three body cavities.

It has homoeostatic effects on all body functions and treats the disorders along the channel.

Ear disorders	—	T.H. 3, T.H. 17, T.H. 21
Dwarfism, Diabetes **(to increase the height), (endocrine point)**	—	T.H. 20
Constipation	—	T.H. 6
Frozen shoulder	—	T.H. 14
Headache	—	T.H. 5, T.H. 23

11. Gall Bladder Channel

Route — It is a Yang channel. **Organ time** - 11.00 pm - 1.00 am

It starts from the head and runs till the foot along the side of the body. It starts from the corner of the eyes, descends down to the neck, again takes a zigzag path over the body, then travels

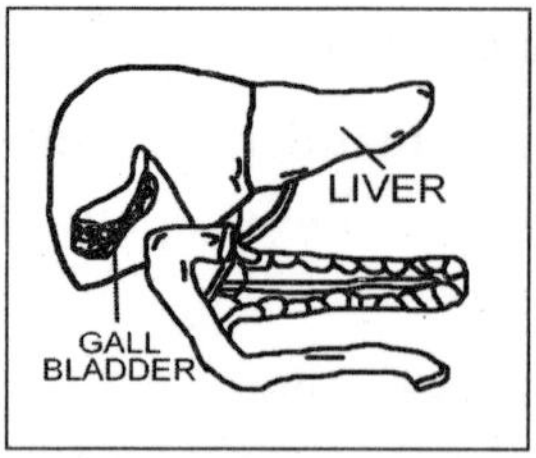

along the side of the leg and ends in the foot at the lateral corner of the 4th toe nail.

Gall bladder stores and secretes bile which is produced by the liver. It is connected to brain. Gall bladder along with the heart has the ability to aid in making decisions and enables clarity in thought.

The channel takes a long route over a number of important regions of the body like eye, ear, brain, neck, breast, liver, gall bladder and sciatic nerve areas. Thus it treats a variety of disorders.

Connection — It is connected to liver channel.

Disharmony — Eye disorders, parietal headache, bitter taste, pain along the pathway of the channel, poor gait, sighing.

It has 44 acupressure points

The commonly used ones are G.B. 1, 2, 8, 14, 20, 21, 24, 25, 26, 30, 31, 34, 40 and 41.

G.B. 1 — 0.5 chun lateral to the outer corner of the eye.
— Eye disorders.

G.B. 2 — In the depression in front of the notch of the ear, easily located when the mouth is open.
— Ear disorders, jaw dislocation, facial paralysis.

G.B. 8 — 1.5 chun over the apex of the ear.
Ear diseases, headache, melancholy.

G.B. 14 — 1 chun over the apex of the eyebrow.
— Eye disorders, frontal headache, sinusitis.

G.B. 20 — 3 chun behind the starting of the ear lobe in the depression.
— Occipital headache, stiff neck, cervical spondylosis, common cold, fever.

G.B. 21 — On the midpoint of the shoulder blade.

— **A special alarm point of the gall bladder, an endocrine point. Useful for treating diabetes,** pain in the shoulder, stiff neck, excessive bleeding during menstruation, miscarriages.

G.B. 24 — Below the nipple on the space between 7th and 8th ribs.

— **Front alarm point of gall bladder.**

Liver diseases (hepatitis) hiccough, gastritis.

G.B. 25 — At the free end of the 12th rib.

— **Alarm point of the kidney,** abdominal distension, pain in the hip joint, nephritis.

G.B. 26 — At the level of the navel, directly below the free end of 11th rib.

— Useful for gynaecological problems, pelvic disorders, back pain, vaginal disorders, vaginal prolapse.

G.B. 30 — On the side of the hip, midpoint to the starting of the lower limb.

— Disorders of the hip joint, sciatica, dislocated lumbar disc, painful thigh, paralysis of the limb.

G.B. 31 — In an erect or lying down position this point lies at the tip of the middle finger when the hand is stretched to side of the thigh.

— Pain or paralysis in the leg, sciatica.

G.B.34 — In the depression below the knee joint along the side.

— **Influential point for muscle and tendons.** Useful for muscle and tendon disorders, disease of the gall bladder, extreme pain in the leg and knee.

G.B. 36 — 7 chun above the tip of the ankle bone on the anterior border of the fibula.

— 7, Sciatica pain and paralysis of the leg.

Gall Bladder Channel

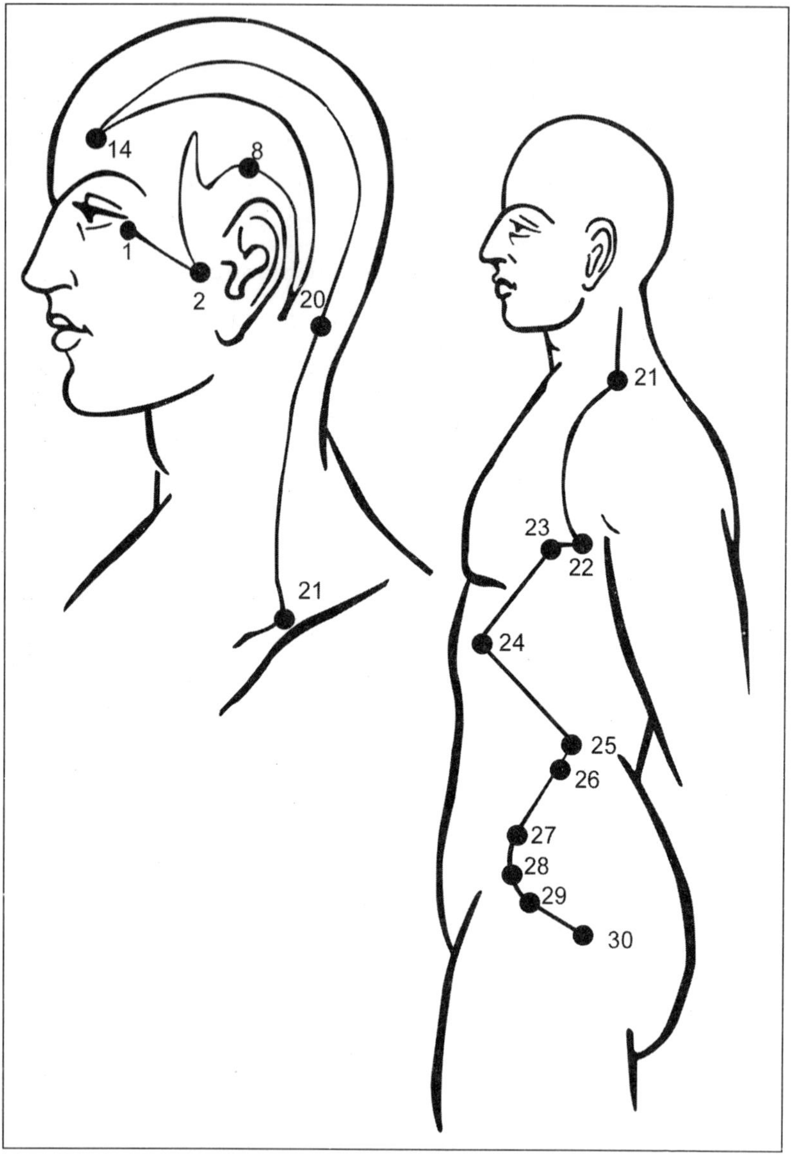

Gall Bladder Channel

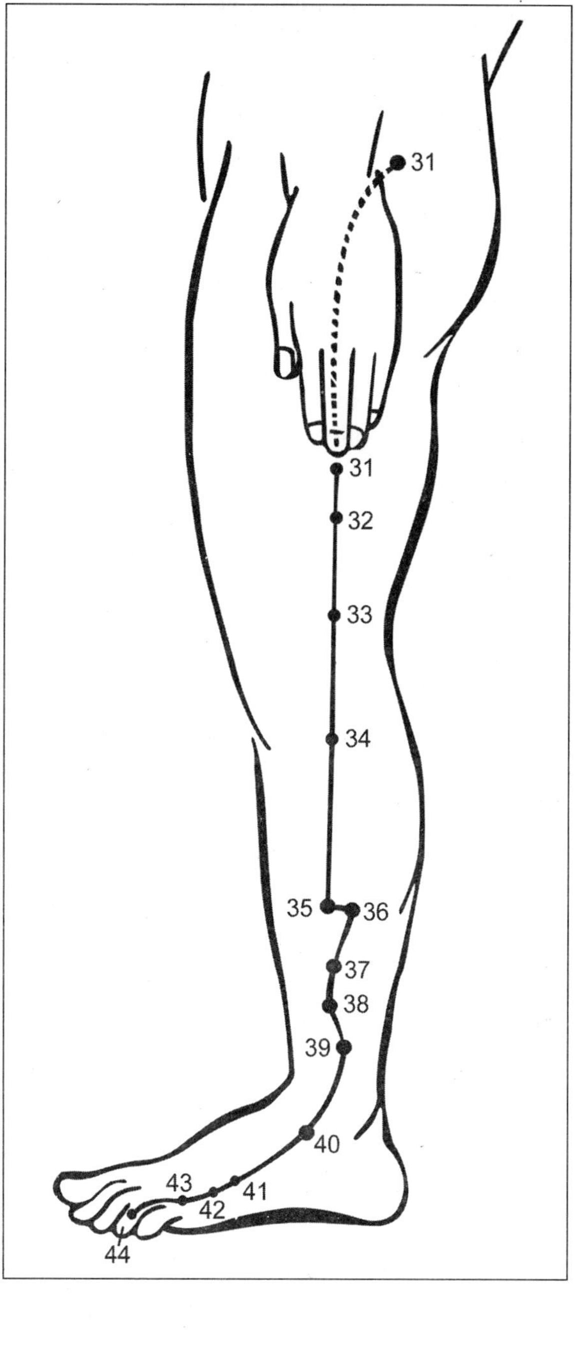

G.B. 37 — 5 chun above the tip of the ankle bone on the anterior border of fibula.

— **It is the connecting point to liver.** Effective for all eye diseases. Muscular pain in the legs.

G.B. 39 — 3 chun above the tip of the ankle bone on the posterior border of fibula.

— **Influential point for bone marrow.** Disorders of the marrow, pain or paralysis of the lower limbs, stiff neck.

G.B. 40 — At the meeting point of two lines, one drawn vertically along the outer border of the ankle, other horizontally along the ankle base.

— **It is a source point.** Ankle disorders, pain in the chest, sciatica, pain in the lower limbs.

G.B. 41 — In the depression at the base of 4th and 5th metatarsals.

— Pain in the foot, ear disorders, painful breast, excessive perspiration.

Source Point	—	G.B. 40
Connection Point	—	G.B. 37
Xi Cleft Point	—	G.B. 36

Five element points		
G.B.44	—	Dryness point
G.B.43	—	Water po int
G.B.41	**—**	**Wind point**
G.B.38	—	Heat point
G.B.34	—	Earth point

The channel has a long course. Starting from the corner of the eye it traverses all over the head, neck, abdomen, thigh, leg and ends at the corner of the small toe.

Use of the points		
Eye disorder	—	G.B. 1
Ear disorder	—	G.B. 2
Migraine, headaches	—	G.B. 8, G.B. 14
Endocrine dysfunctioning (diabetes)	—	G.B. 21

To check gall bladder disorders	—	G.B. 24
To check kidney disorder	—	G.B. 25
Hip joint disorder and leg pain	—	G.B. 30, G.B. 31, G.B. 36
Muscle and tendon weakness	—	G.B. 34
Bone marrow disorders	—	G.B. 39

12. Liver Channel

Route — It is a Yin channel. **Organ time** — 1.00 am - 3.00 am

It starts from the big toe, runs along the upper part of the foot, climbs up the leg along the inner side, circles round genitals, takes a diagonal route along the abdomen and reaches the chest and ends below the nipple in the space between 6th and 7th ribs.

Liver discharges bile. It stimulates digestion. It is responsible for storage and release of the blood. When body is at rest it stops the blood and releases during activity. It is sensitive to emotional changes. The effects are felt bothways. Liver upset results in frustration, irritability, stress, anger, shouting, hysteria, violence, Prevalence of these emotions can also affect the liver.

Liver is involved in menstrual disorders and sexual problems as the meridian encircles the genitals.

Liver is the spring of the body. It has strong upward movement. An overactive liver leads to hyperactivity, explosive temper, splitting headache, nose bleeds, bitter taste in the mouth.

Because of its connection to gall bladder it is also effective for mental disorders, headache, etc.

Connection — Liver is connected to gall bladder channel.

Importance — Liver **governs** muscles and tendons.

— Liver **opens** to the eyes. The **colour** of the nails turn greenish on malfunctioning of the liver. The liver is connected to **Element:** wood, **Colour:** green, **Emotion:** anger, **Sound:** shouting.

Disharmony — Pain along the channel, fullness of chest, weak vision, vertical headache, dizziness.

It has 14 acupressure points

The commonly used ones are Liv. 3, 6, 8, 13 and 14.

Liv. 3 — 2 chun from the web of 1st and 2nd toes.

— **It is source point. It is a good homoeostatic point.**

Liver Channel

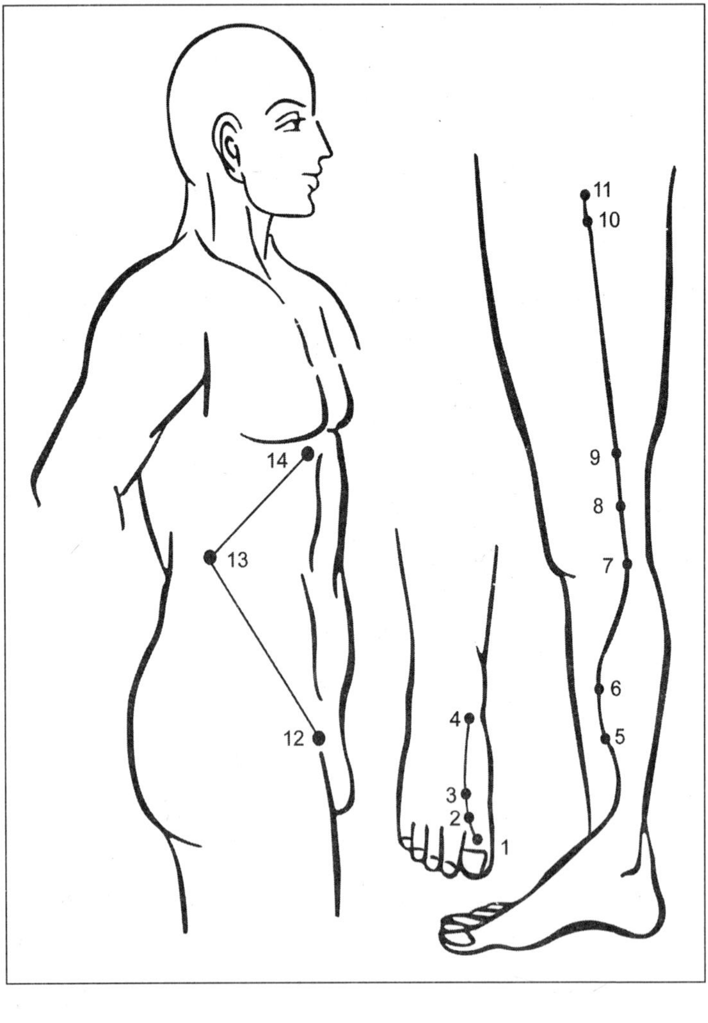

— Eye disease, hypertension (blood pressure), headaches, diarrhoea, constipation, difficulty in walking.

Liv. 6 — 7 chun from the upper end of the ankle joint.

— **It is a xi cleft point. A special alarm point of the liver.**

Liver and gall bladder disorders.

Liv. 8 — In the crease of the knee joint at its inner end.

— Disorders of the knee joint. The point is effective for genital problems. For impotence, irregular menstruation, pain in the penis, to increase sperm count.

Liv. 13 — At the free end of the 11th rib.

— **Influential point for the Yin organs. Alarm point of the spleen.** Disorders of liver and spleen, abdominal swelling, flatulence, strenuous respiration.

Liv. 14 — Below the nipple, in the space between 6th and 7th ribs.

— **Alarm point of liver.**

— Chest pain, coughing, belching, vomiting, hepatitis.

Source Point	—	Liv. 3
Connection Point	—	Liv. 5
Xi Cleft Point	—	Liv. 6

Five element points		
Liv.1	—	**Wind point**
Liv.2	—	Heat point
Liv.3	—	Earth point
Liv.4	—	Dryness point
Liv.8	—	Water point

Liver channel influences gastro-urinary organs, eye problems, muscle and tendon disorders, vertical headaches, blood pressure, etc.

Use of points		
Eye disorder	—	Liv. 2
Blood disorder	—	Liv. 3
(a good homoeostatic point)		

Impotence	—	Liv. 8
To check liver and gall bladder disorders	—	Liv. 6, Liv. 13
Headache	—	Liv. 2, Liv. 5

13. Du Channel (Governing Vessel Channel)

Route — It is a Yang channel.

It starts from just below the coccyx, moves up over the spinal cord and the brain, descends over the forehead, down the nose and ends just above the lips.

This is an unpaired channel. It has governing or controlling influence over all other Yang channels.

The channel runs over the spinal cord and the brain. Hence its functions are closely linked to the central nervous system.

It has 28 acupressure points

The commonly used ones are Du. 1, 3, 4, 6, 11, 14, 15, 16, 20, 23, 25, 26 and 28.

Du. 1 — Midpoint between tip of the coccyx and the anus.

It is connecting point to Ren. 1.

— Haemorrhoids, rectal prolapse, low backache, wind in large intestine, itching of anus, impotence.

Du. 3 — On the spinal cord between 4th and 5th lumbar vertebrae, just above the buttocks.

— Low backache, genito-urinary disorders, impotence, abdominal distension.

Du. 4 — On the spinal cord between 2nd and 3rd lumbar vertebrae.

— Low backache, genito-urinary disorders, impotence.

Du. 6 — On the spinal cord between 11th and 12th thoracic vertebrae.

Governing Vessel Channel

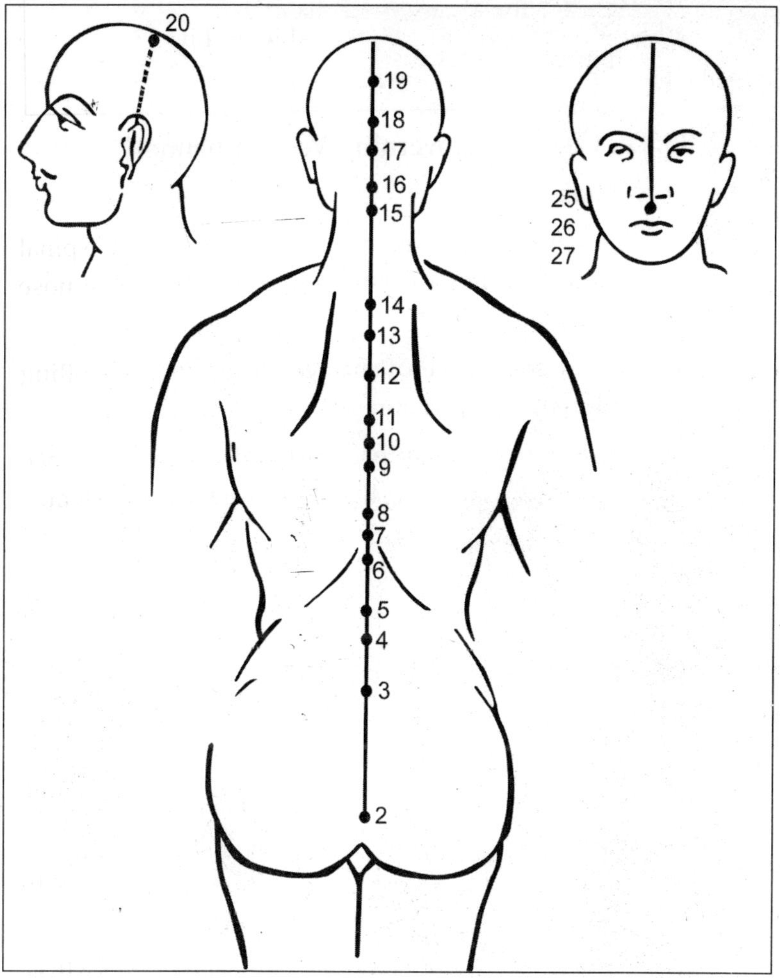

— Epilepsy, insanity, abdomen distended, this point causes muscular relaxation in spastic states.

Du. 11 — On the spinal cord between 5th and 6th thoracic vertebrae.

— Cardiac diseases, nervousness, loss of memory, incoherent speech.

Du. 14 — On the spinal cord between the 7th thoracic vertebra and 1st thoracic vertebra.

— **It is very important immune enhancing point.** It is used for a variety of disorders.

Immune disorders	—	Fever, cold, infections.
Mental disorders	—	Epilepsy, headache, migraine, nervousness.
Local disorders	—	Cervical spondylosis, Frozen shoulder.
Lung disorders	—	Asthma, bronchitis, severe cough.

Du. 15 — 0.5 chun above the back hairline between 1st and 2nd thoracic vertebrae.

— **It is a very sensitive and dangerous point.**

Deaf mutism, speech difficulties, complete or partial loss of voice.

Du. 16 — 1 chun above the back hairline along the spinal cord.

— **This is also a sensitive and dangerous point.**

Headache, deafness and dumbness, mental disorders, stiff neck, nose block, cerebral haemorrhage.

Du. 20 — 5 chun behind the front hairline. It can also be traced by drawing a line from the apex of the ear and at the point where it meets the midline.

— It is the meeting point of a number of points. **It is a very good sedative and tranquillising point.**

— It is used for treating a variety of disorders, **mental disorders** — epilepsy, insomnia, Parkinsonism, schizophrenia, insanity, severe fright, all conditions where psychogenic factors exist, bronchial asthma, impotence, headache, loss of memory, falling of head hair, rectal prolapse (used here as a distal point).

Du. 23 — 1 chun above the midpoint of the front hairline.

— Nose block, headache, face red and swollen.

Du. 25 — At the tip of the nose.

— Nose block, sores inside nose, bulbous nose from drinking excess alcohol.

Du. 26 — In the space between the nose and the lip along the midline. This point lies in distance between upper 1/3rd and lower 2/3rd of nose and the lip.

— Here 3 Yang channels meet. **An emergency point for Yang depleted problems.** Fainting, epileplsy, hysteria, heatstroke, acute low backache (used here as a distal point), facial paralysis, swelling in the face, excessive thirst.

Connection point	—	Du. 1

It is the governing vessel meridian. Governs the functions of other meridians.

Use of Points		
Low backache, genito-urinary disorders, impotence	—	Du. 3, Du. 4
Immune disorders, (fever, skin troubles)	—	Du. 14, Du. 20
Neurological problems (epilepsy)	—	Du. 4, Du. 20
Emergency situations (fainting, fits, heatstroke)	—	Du. 26

14. Ren Channel (Conception Vessel)

Route — It is a Yin channel. It is a Yin channel.

It starts from the centre of the perineum and moves up along the midline in front of the body, over the abdomen, chest, neck and ends just below the lips.

It is an important channel and helps in various reproductive problems, hence the name conception vessel. **It has 6 alarm**

points along its route indicating and rectifying the problems in a number of vital organs of the body.

It has 24 acupressure points

The commonly used ones are Ren. 1, 2, 3, 4, 5, 6, 9, 12, 17, 22, 23, and 24.

Ren. 1 — In the centre of perineum.

— All diseases of the perineum area. Pain in vagina, vagina swollen, painful, irregular periods, penis painful, prolapse of vagina, haemorrhoids.

Ren. 2 — On the midpoint just above pubic border.

— Genito-urinary disorders.

Menstrual disorders, impotence, lack of virility, spermatorrhoea, incontinence and retention of urine, lower abdomen swollen.

Ren. 3 — 4 chun below navel.

— **Alarm point of urinary bladder.**

Genito-urinary disorders, same as Ren. 2.

Fibroids, excessive vaginal discharge, general fatigue.

Ren. 4 — 3 chun below navel.

— **Alarm point of small intestine.**

— Genito-urinary disorders, same as Ren. 2.

— Also diarrhoea, retained placenta.

Ren. 5 — 2 chun below the navel.

— **Alarm point of Triple heater.**

Oedema, ascites, abdomen swollen, food not digested, general fatigue.

Ren. 6 — 1.5 chun below the navel.

— **This is a good tonification point.**

Used for chronic fatigue, hypertension, insomnia.

Ren. 8 — In the centre of the navel.

— Diarrhoea, swollen abdomen, fainting and various Yin disorders.

Ren. 9 — 1 chun above navel.

Conception Vessel

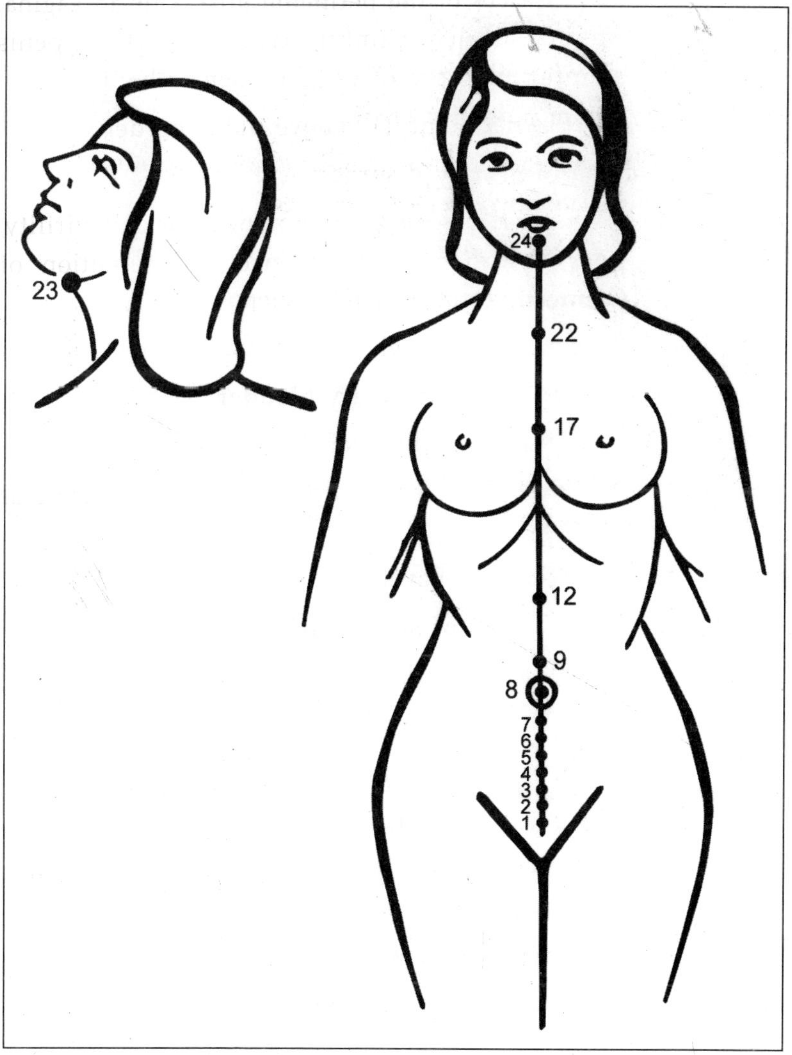

— **Specific point for oedema,** swollen abdomen, flatulence.

Ren. 12 — 4 chun above the navel.

— **Alarm point for stomach. Influential point for all Yang organs. Union point for five Yang organs.** All gastric disorders, nausea, vomiting, abdominal distension, flatulence, peptic ulcer, stomach pain, acute gastroenteritis.

Ren. 14 — 6 chun above the navel.

— **Alarm point for heart.**

— Chest painful, cardiac pain, fainting, confusion and melancholy, mental illnesses.

Ren. 15 — 7 chun above the navel along the midline.

— **Connecting point of vital centres.**

— Cardiac disease, palpitation, insanity, walks around wildly and restlessly, vomiting, gastric pain.

Ren. 17 — On the sternum midway between the two nipples.

— **Alarm point of the pericardium. Influential point for respiratory system.**

— All lung diseases. Bronchial asthma, severe cough, heart and chest painful, breast disorders.

Ren. 22 — 0.5 chun above the U-notch in the neck.

— Dry cough, bronchial asthma, throat swollen, sores in throat which prevent eating, goitre.

Ren. 23 — In the midline of the neck, midway between Adam's apple and the chin.

— Difficulty in speaking, mutism, stammering, excessive salivation, sores in mouth, throat constricted, pharyngitis, laryngitis.

Ren. 24 — In the middle of the chin along the midline.

— Facial paralysis, face swollen, toothache, dental caries, swelling of gums, dumbness.

Connection point — Ren. 15

As the name implies the meridian helps in reproductive function and controls all Yin channels.

Use of Points

Genital problems, impotence, spermatorrhoea, menstrual problems, chronic inflammation	—	Ren. 2, Ren. 3, Ren. 4
Tonification of the lower abdominal organs	—	Ren. 6
Nausea, vomiting, peptic ulcer, gas problems	—	Ren. 12
Oedema	—	Ren. 8, Ren. 9
Respiratory problem	—	Ren. 17
Toothache, swelling in gums	—	Ren. 24

The Starting and Ending of Channels are at the Finger Tips and Toe Ends

These are vital points for stimulation. They have storewell of energy belonging to the particular channel.

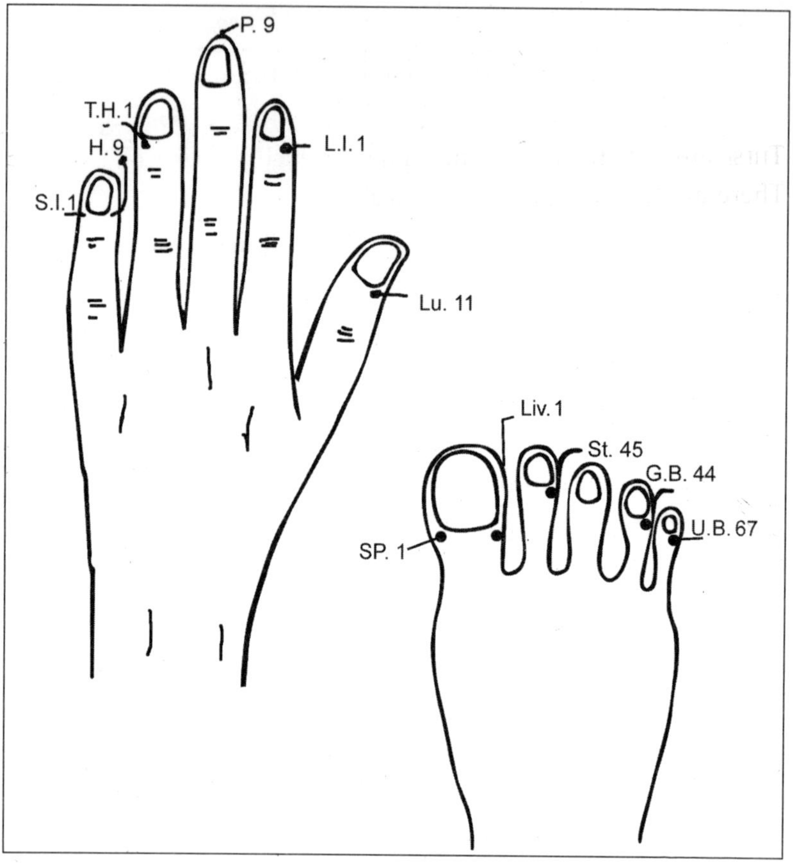

8

Influential Points

THESE are specific acupuncture points which treat specific tissues. There are in all eight influential points.

Tissues	Points
Respiratory tissues	Ren. 17
Bone and cartilage	U.B. 11
Blood	U.B. 17
Hollow (Yang) organs	Ren. 12
Solid (Yin) organs	Liv. 13
Vascular organs	Lu. 9
Muscle and tendon	G.B. 34
Bone marrow	G.B. 39

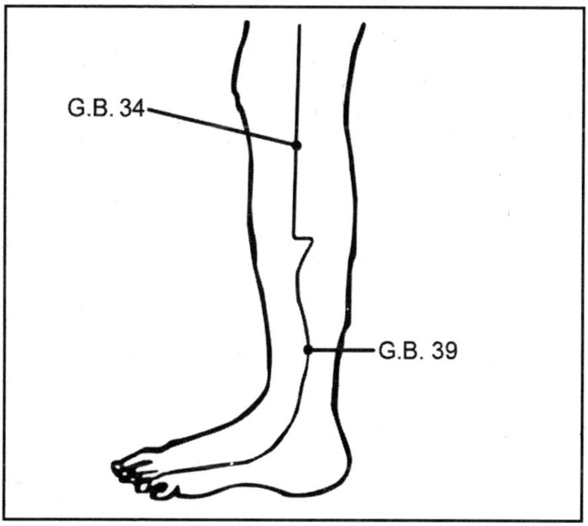

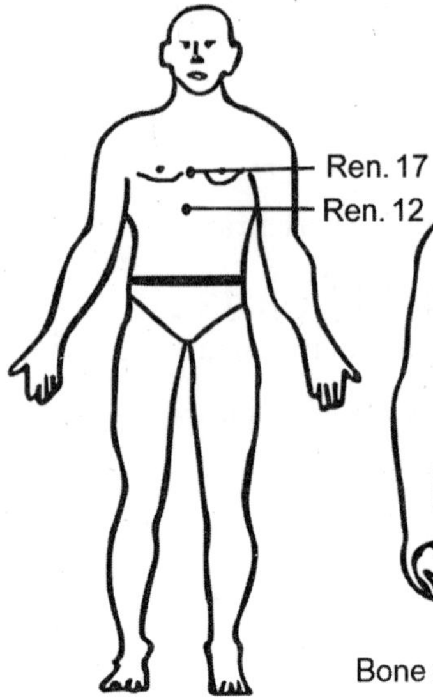

Respiratory Tissues- Ren. 17
Hollow (Yang) organs- Ren. 12

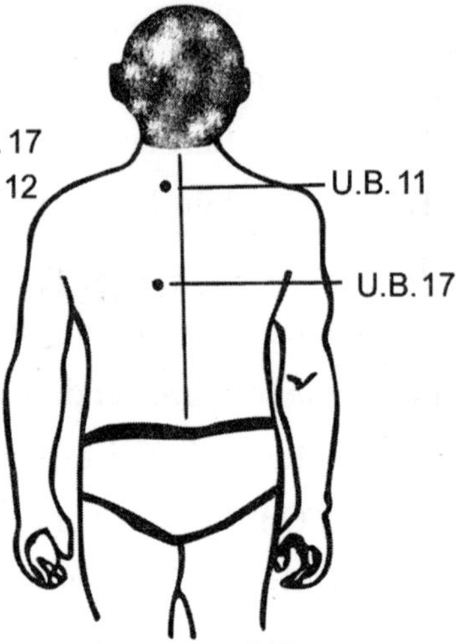

Bone and cartilage- U.B. 11
Blood U.B. 17

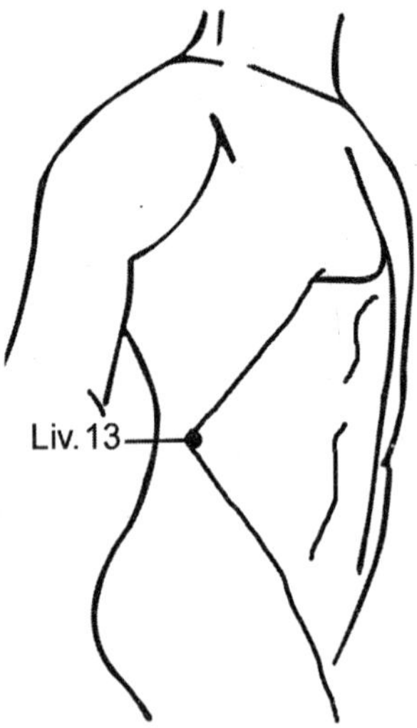

Solid (Yin) organs- Liv. 13

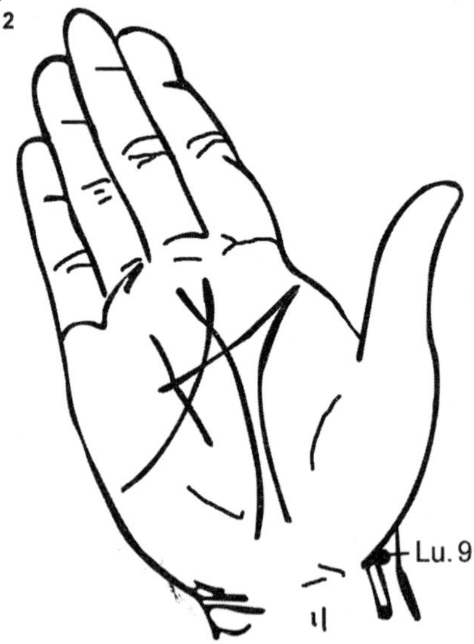

Vascular Organ

Ren. 17 — On the midline of the sternum, midway between the two nipples.

Represented as pericardium alarm pt.

U.B. 11 — 1.5 chun lateral to 1st vertebra.

U.B. 17 — 1.5 chun lateral to 7th vertebra.

Ren. 12 — 4 chun above the navel.

— Represented as stomach alarm pt.

Liv. 13 — At the free end of the 11th rib.

— Represented as spleen alarm pt.

Lu. 9 — On the outer end of wrist crease.

G.B. 34 — On the outer surface of the lower leg below fibula head.

G.B. 39 — On the outer surface of the lower leg 3 chun above ankle joint.

Distal Point

The pressure points located in distal places, away from the location of trouble help at times effectively in treating the disorders.

This is because the energy through the channel reaches the point of trouble.

There are six important distal points, three in the leg and three in the hand.

The Distal Points of the Hand

Distal Point	*Area Effective*
L.I. 4	Face, sense organs in the face, front of the head and neck.
Lu. 7	Back of the head and neck, back of the chest and lungs.
P. 6	Front of the chest, internal organs of chest, diaphragm.

Distal Points of the Hand

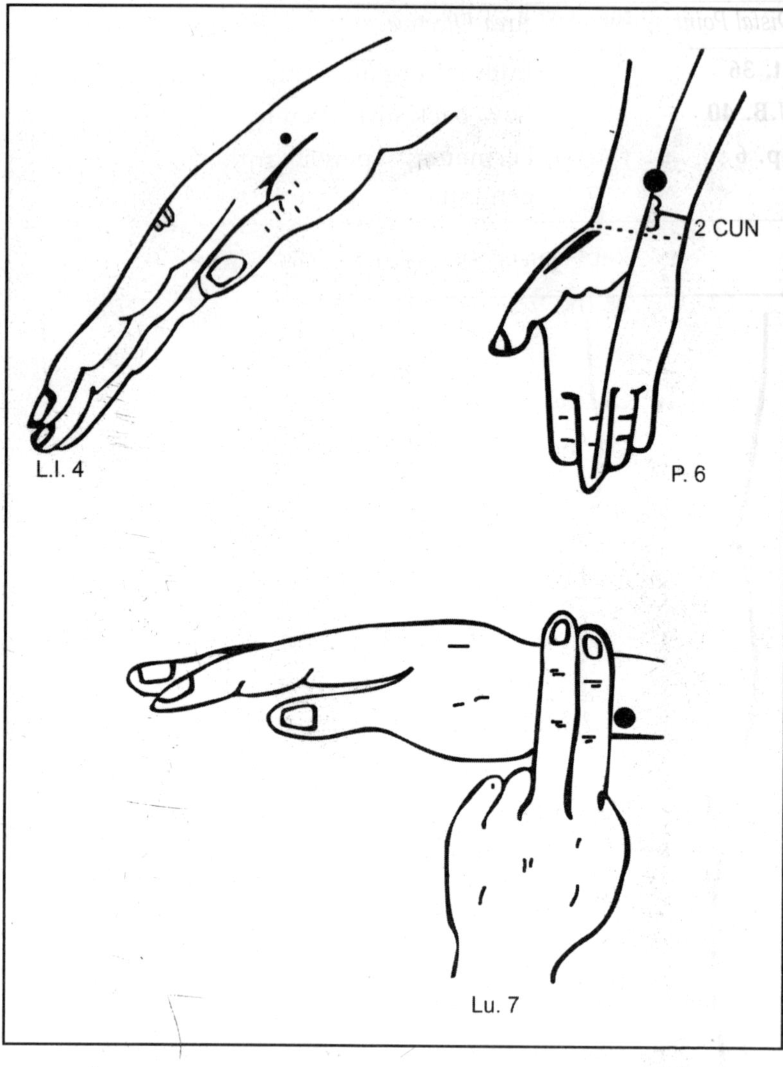

The Distal Points of the Leg

Distal Point	*Area Effective*
St. 36	Internal organs of the abdomen.
U.B. 40	Low back, urinogenital organs.
Sp. 6	Perineum, pelvic organs, external genitalia.

Distal Points of the Leg

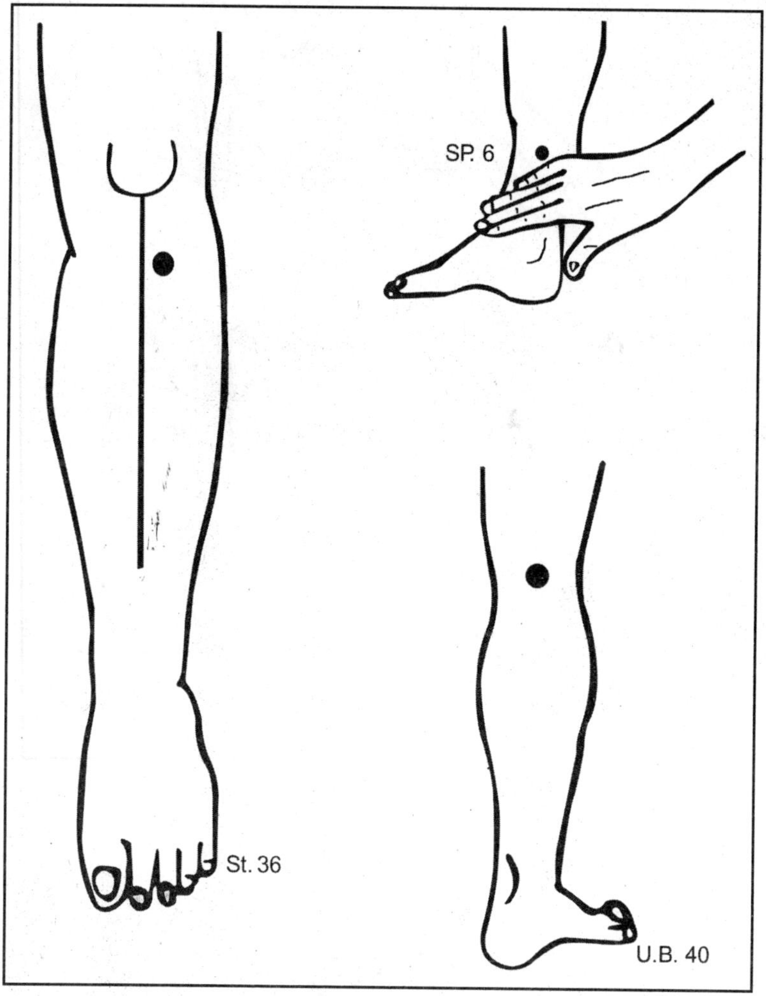

Specific Effect Points

On stimulating certain points specific effects are produced.

They are —

Analgesic (pain removing) — L.I. 4, St. 43, St. 44.

Analgesic (Pain Removing) Points

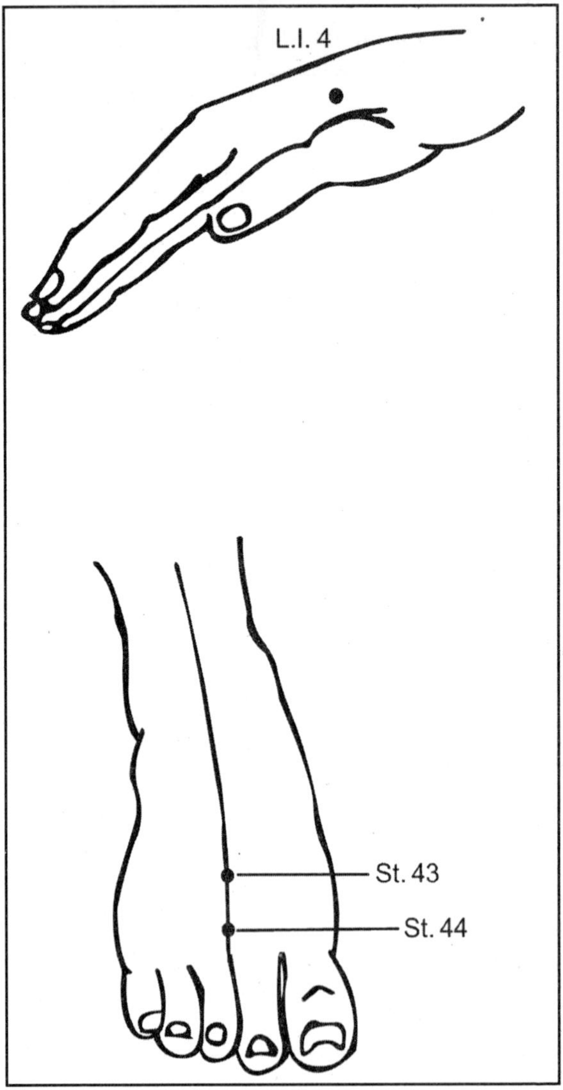

Sedative Points

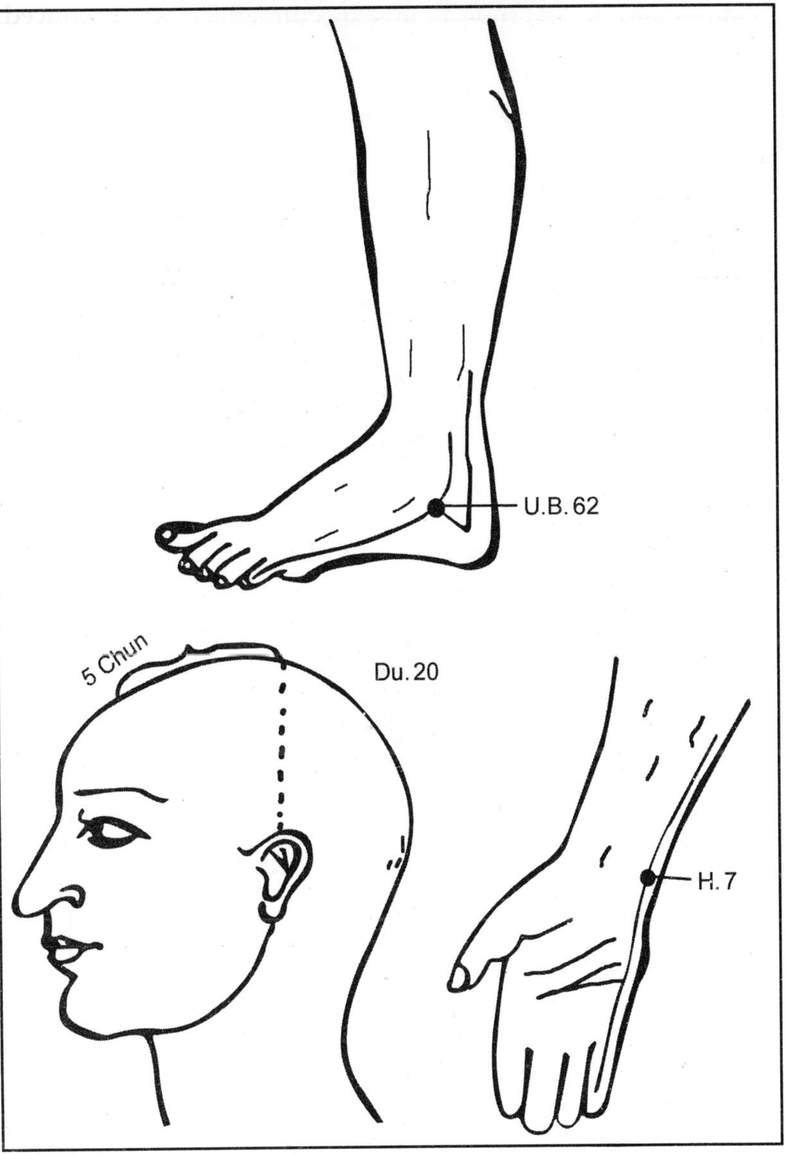

Homoeostasis Points

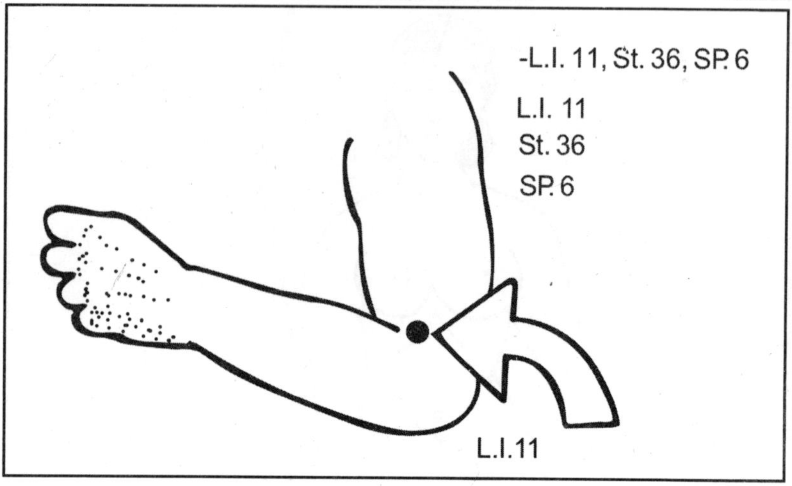

Immune Enhancing

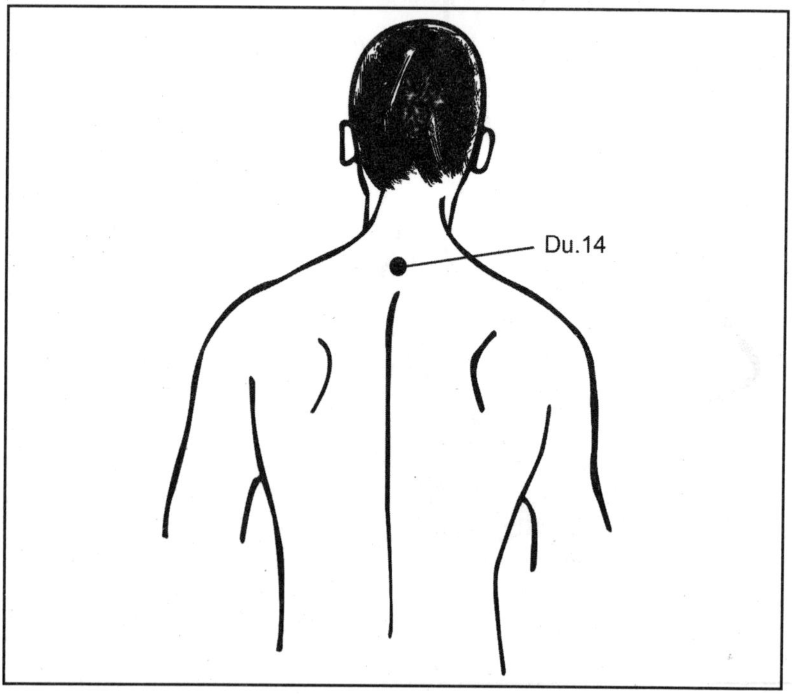

Tonification

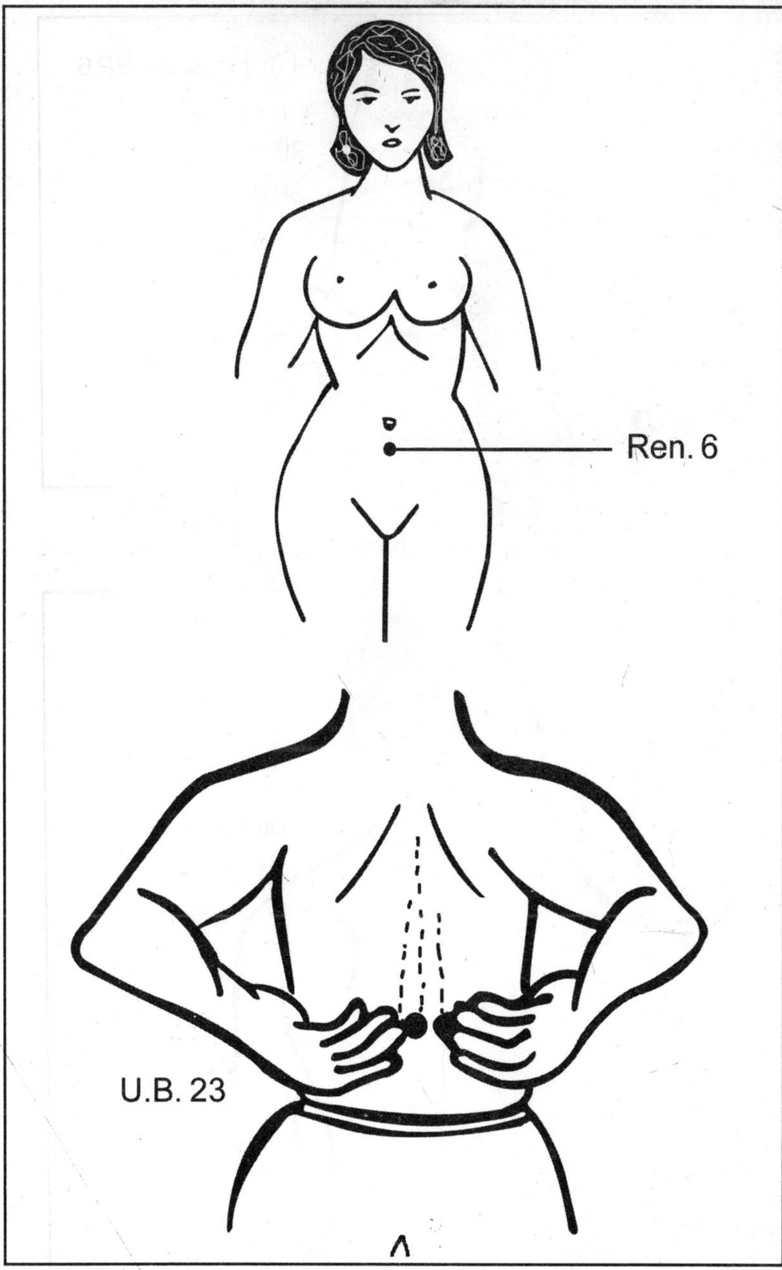

Emergency Points

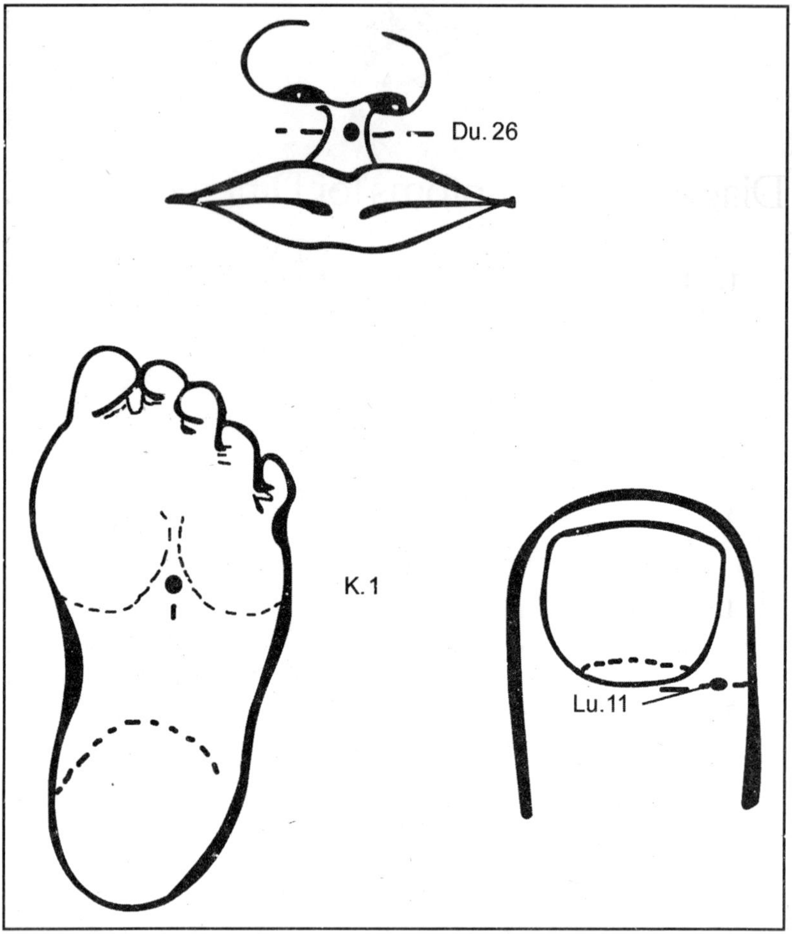

9

Diagnosing Symptoms for Different Organs

1. **Lung** — Cough, fullness of chest, bronchial asthma, pharyngitis, pain along the course of the channel.
2. **Large Intestine** — Pain along the channel, sore throat, swelling of the cheek, frozen shoulder, pharyngitis, tooth-ache.
3. **Heart** — Pain along the medial aspect of the upper limb, night sweating, dryness of the throat.
4. **Small Intestine** — Pain along the channel, sore throat, swelling of the cheek, deafness, lower abdominal pain.
5. **Stomach** — Mental disturbance, deviation of the eyes and mouth, sore throat, pain in the chest and abdomen, pain and paralysis of the anterior aspect of the lower limb and dorsum of the foot.
6. **Spleen** — Erection of gas from the stomach (belching), nausea, vomiting, pain at the root of the tongue.
7. **Pericardium** — Symptoms same as those of heart.
8. **Triple Heater** — Pain along the channel and ear disorders.
9. **Urinary Bladder** — Uneasiness when exposed to wind. Vertical and occipital headache, backache and sciatic.
10. **Kidney** — Lack of energy, low backache, dark circles under eyes, tinnitus, irregular menstruation.

11. **Liver** — Lower abdominal symptoms and pain in genitals. Frigidity and impotence may also result.

12. **Gall Bladder Channel** — Eye disorders, parietal headache, bitter taste, pain along the pathway of the channel.

10

Diseases and Relevant Points Used for Treatment

Respiratory Disorders

Lung, Du and Ren. channels are commonly used.

Alarm Pt of Lungs	—	Lu. 1 (front alarm point), U.B. 13 (back alarm point)
Common cold	—	Du. 14, Du. 20, Lu. 6
Cough	—	Lu. 7, Ren. 22, Ren. 17
Asthmatic attack	—	Lu. 6, Ren. 22, Ren. 17, Du. 20, U.B. 13
(asthmatic emergency	—	To prick Lu. 11 during attack)
Sinusitis	—	G.B. 14, S.I. 18, U.B. 2, L.I. 11
Tonsillitis	—	S.I. 17, L.I. 4, Du. 20, Du. 14
Hoarse voice	—	Ren. 23, L.I. 18, S.I. 17, Du. 14
Blocked nose	—	L.I. 19, L.I. 20
Nosebleeding	—	Du. 23, Du. 26, L.I. 19 U.B. 17 (Influential point for blood)

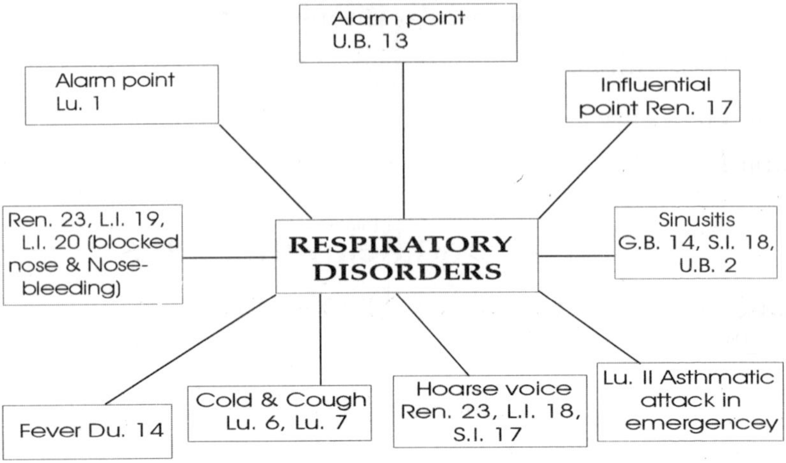

Respiratory Disorders

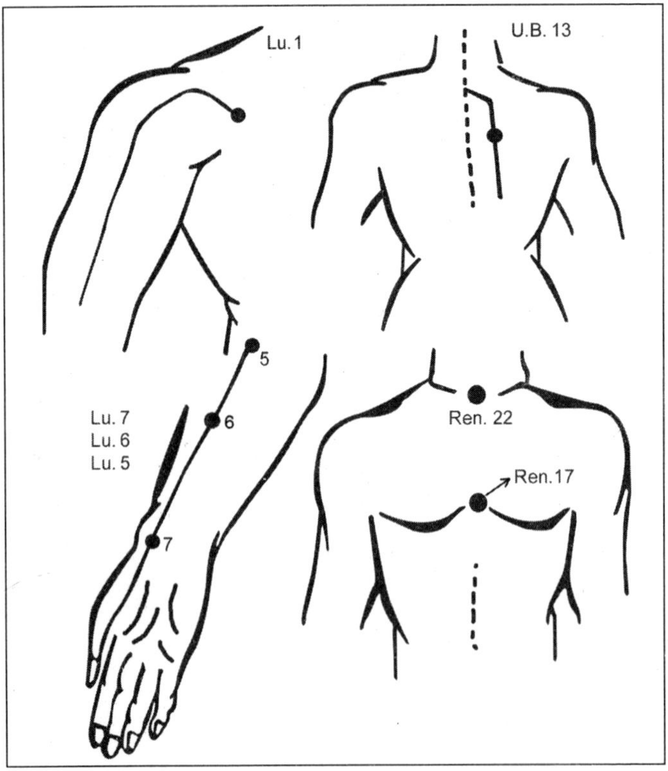

Cardiovascular Disorders

Heart, Pericardium, Ren. channels are commonly used.

Alarm Pt. of Heart — Ren. 14 (front) U.B. 15 (back)

Alarm Pt. of Pericardium — Ren. 17 (front) U.B. 14 (back)

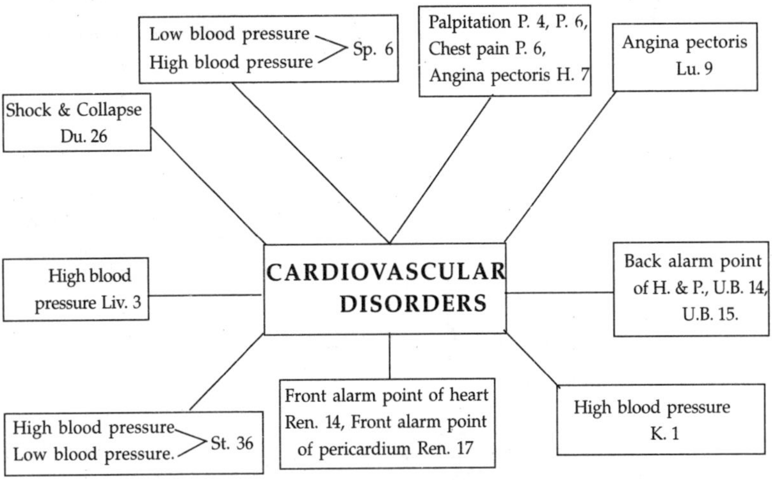

Shock and collapse	—	Du. 26
Palpitation	—	P. 4, P. 6, Du. 20
Insomnia, restlessness	—	H. 7, U.B. 62, Du. 20, Du. 26
Anxiety, Chest pain	—	U.B. 15, U.B. 14, P. 6, L.I. 4
Low blood pressure	—	Ren. 6, St. 36, Sp. 6
High blood pressure	—	Du. 20, L.I. 11, St. 36, Sp. 6, Liv. 3, K. 1
Angina pectoris	—	Ren. 17, U.B. 15, P..6, H. 7, Lu. 9, Du. 20
Blood disorder (Ex: anaemia)	—	U.B. 17, Ren. 6, Sp. 6, G.B. 39

Cardiovascular Disorders

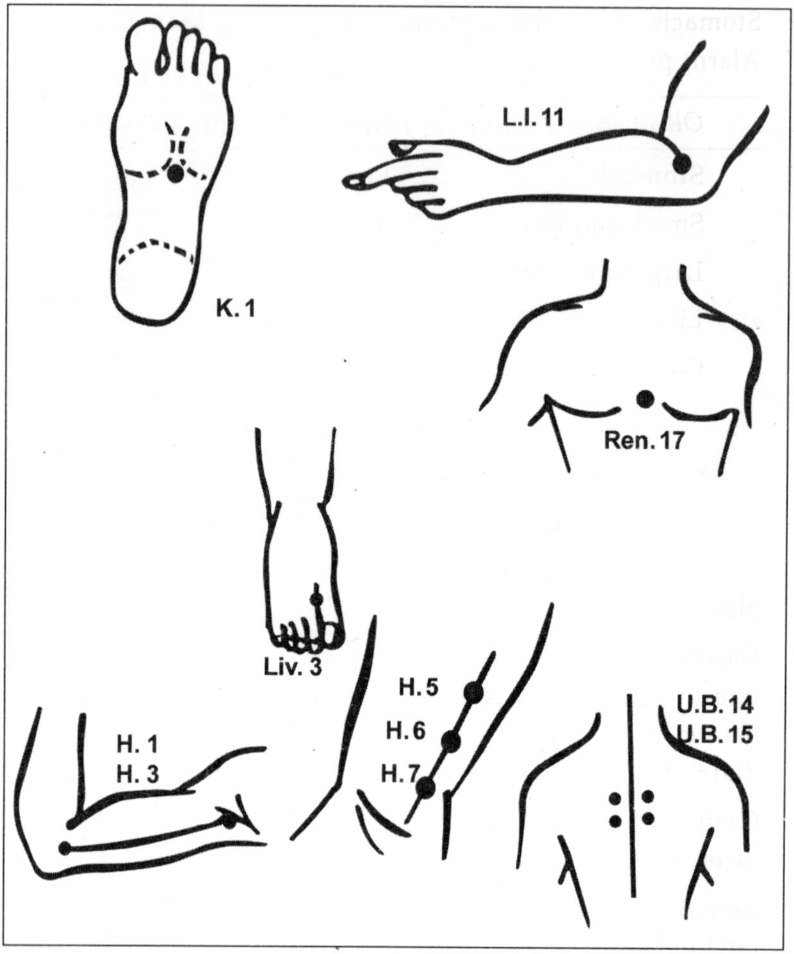

Gastrointestinal Disorders

Stomach, Ren and Spleen channels are commonly used, Alarm pt. for gastrointestinal organs.

ORGANS	*FRONT A.P.*	*BACK A.P.*
Stomach	Ren. 12	U.B. 21
Small intestine	Ren. 4	U.B. 27
Large intestine	St. 25	U.B. 25
Liver	Liv. 6	U.B. 18
Gall bladder	Ex. 35	U.B. 19
	G.B. 21	
	G.B. 24	
Spleen	Liv. 13	U.B. 20
Appendix	Liv. 33	

Nausea and vomiting	P. 6, Ren. 12, Liv. 13, Du. 20
Gastritis (inflammation of the intestinal lining leading to nausea, vomiting, fever and diarrhoea)	St. 34, St. 36, St. 35, Ren. 12 Sp. 6, P. 6
Gastric ulcer, duodenal ulcer, peptic ulcer	St. 21, St. 25, U.B. 20, U.B. 21, Ren. 12, St. 36, Sp. 6
Indigestion leading to (abdominal distension, nausea, diarrhoea or constipation)	Same as above
Flatulence, gas in stomach	G.B. 25, G.B. 26, Liv. 13, Ren. 12, Ex. 33, St. 36
Appendix	St. 25, St. 29, Ren. 12, Ex. 33, St. 36
Intestinal parasites (Amoebiasis and other worms)	Sp. 15, Sp. 25, Ren. 12, St. 36

Diarrhoea, dysentry	St. 25, Ren. 3, St. 34, St. 36
Constipation	St. 25, St. 36, Sp. 6, Ren. 12
Piles	Du. 1, Ren. 1, U.B. 54, Sp. 6, Du. 6

Ulcer — St. 21, St. 25, Ren. 12

Stomach Alarm Point Ren. 12
Small intestine Alarm point Ren. 4
Stomach Alarm point St. 25

Liver Alarm point Liv. 6

Gas in stomach G.B. 25, G.B. 26, Liv. 13, Ren. 12.

GASTROINTESTINAL DISORDERS

Liver Alarm point U.B. 18
G.B. Alarm point U.B. 19
St. Alarm point U.B. 21
Spleen Alarm point U.B. 20

Nausea, Vomitting Diarrhoea St. 34, St. 36, St. 25, St. 21, Ren. 12.

Small intestine Alarm point U.B. 27
Large intestine Alarm U.B. 25

G.B. Alarm point G.B.21, G.B. 24,
Spleen Alarm point Liv. 13

Gastrointestinal Disorders

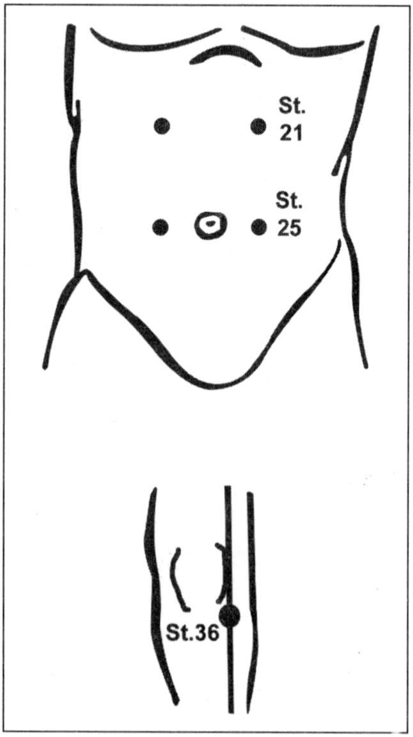

Gastrointestinal Disorders

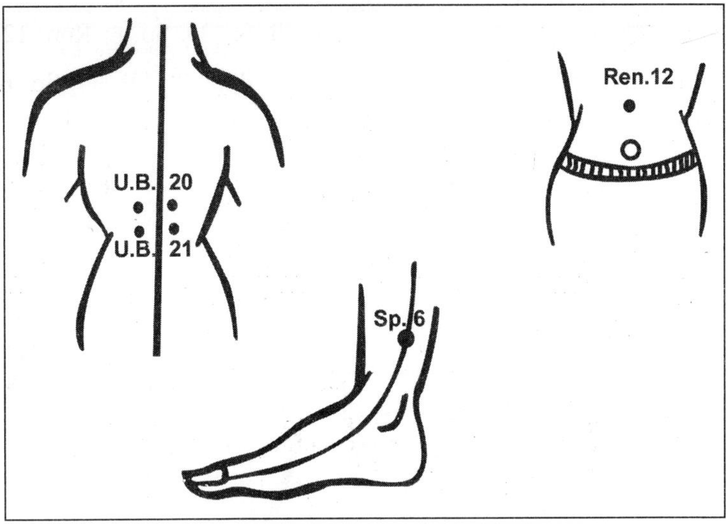

Liver and Spleen Disorders

Liver, gall bladder, spleen and stomach channels are commonly used.

Alarm point of liver	Liv. 14, Liv. 6
Alarm point of spleen	Liv. 13
Alarm point of gall bladder	G.B. 24, G.B. 21, Ex. 35
Jaundice	Liv. 13, Liv. 14, G.B. 24, G.B. 26, Liv. 6, U.B. 19, U.B. 20, U.B. 21, G.B. 34, St. 36, Sp. 6, Ren. 6
Cirrhosis of the liver	Same as above. Sp. 9, Ren. 5, Ren. 9
Gall bladder stone	G.B. 24, Liv. 13, Liv. 14, U.B. 18, U.B. 19, L.I. 4
Enlargement of spleen	Du. 20, Liv. 13, Liv. 14, G.B. 24, G.B. 26, St. 21, U.B. 20

Liver and Spleen Disorders

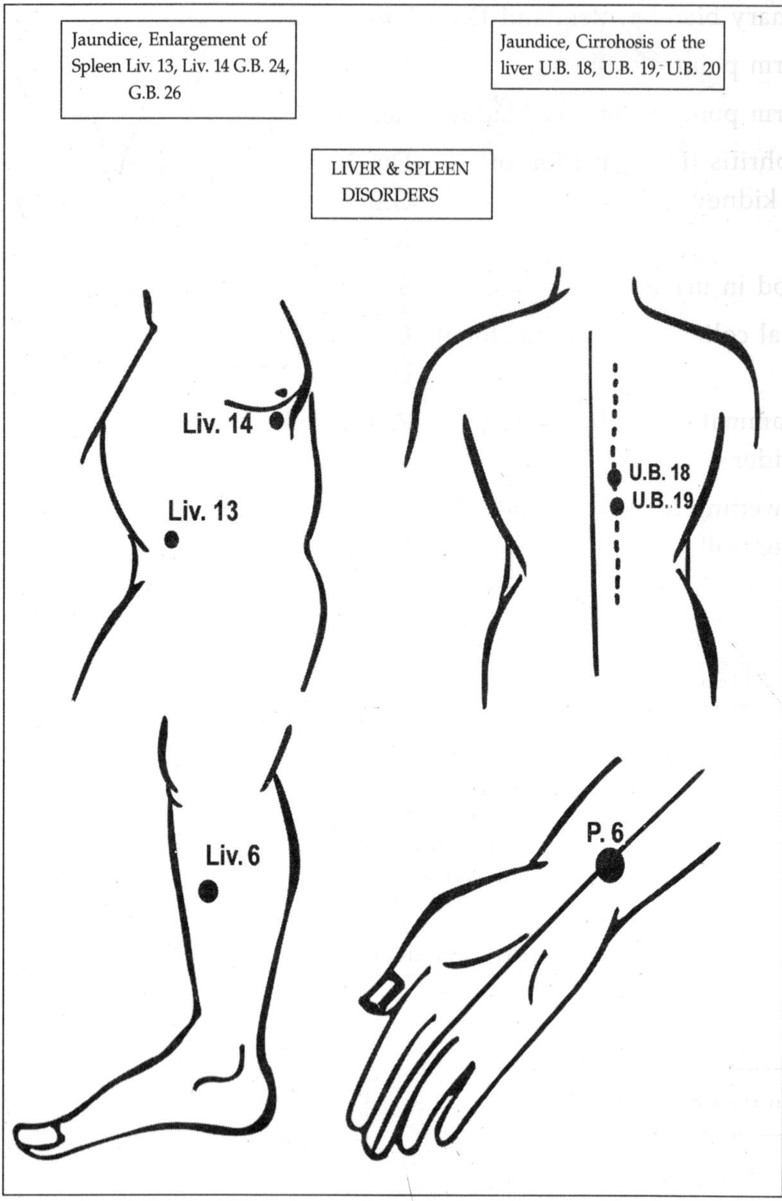

Genito-Urinary Disorders

Urinary bladder, Ren. and Du. Channels are commonly used.

Alarm point of kidney	G.B. 25, U.B. 23
Alarm point of urinary bladder	Ren. 3, U.B. 28
Nephritis (inflammation of the kidney)	Du. 20, U.B. 23, U.B. 25 G.B. 26, Du. 4, Du. 3, Ren. 3, K. 3
Blood in urine	Same as above
Renal colic (often due to stone)	Liv. 4, K. 5, U.B. 23, Du. 2, U.B. 25, U.B. 24, K. 3, P. 6
Inflammation of the urinary bladder	Ren. 3, Ren. 4, U.B. 32, Du. 14, L.I. 11, Sp. 6, Sp. 9, U.B. 40
Bedwetting (due to inability in controlling bladder muscles)	Ren. 3, Ren. 4, U.B. 32, Ren. 6, U.B. 23, K. 3

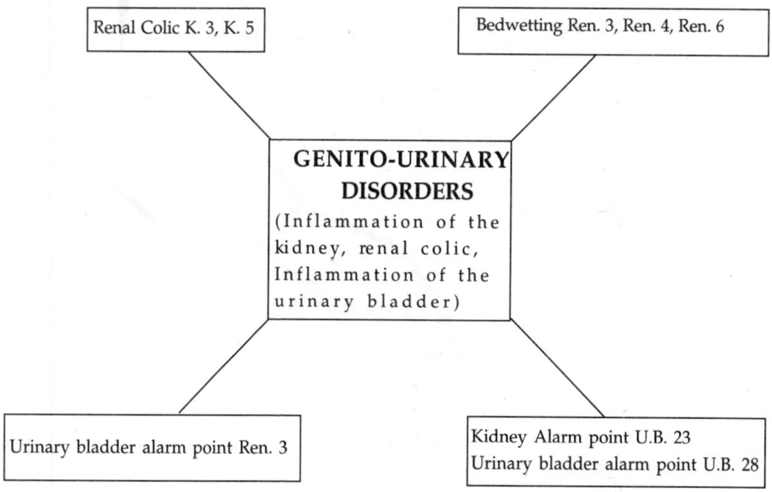

Genito-Urinary Disorders

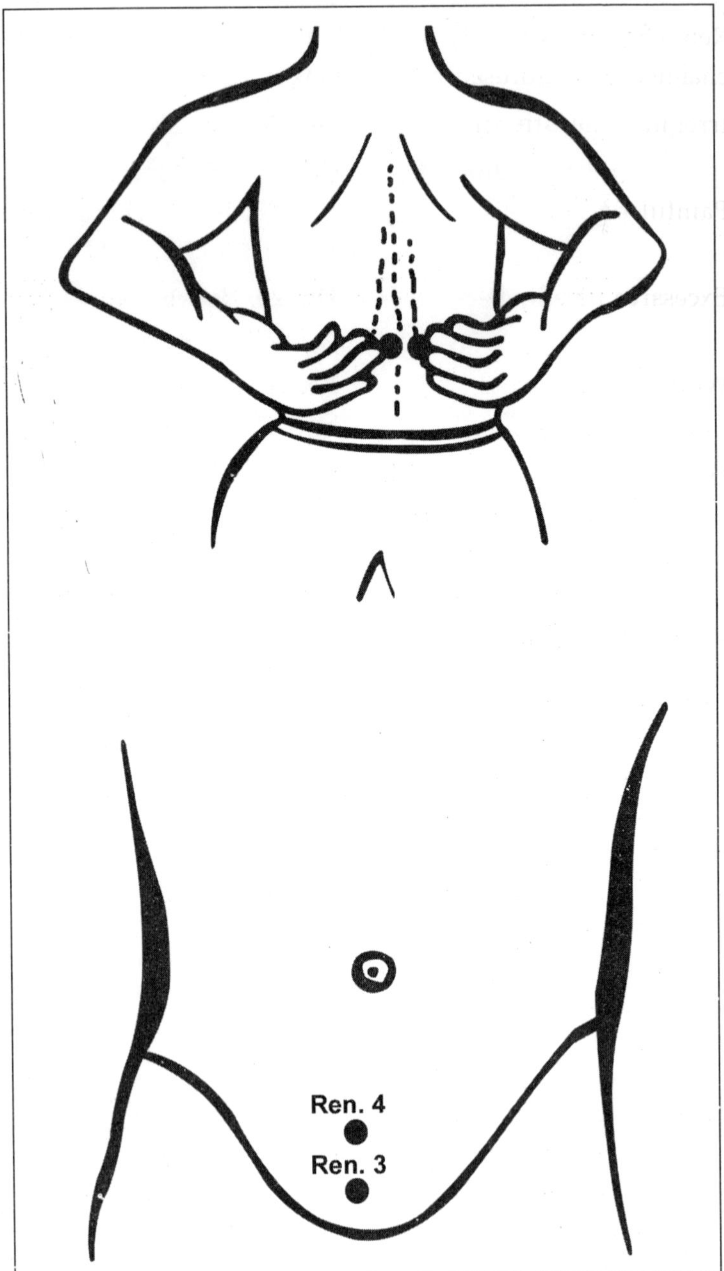

Disorders of Women

Ren. channel is mostly used. Stomach, spleen, urinary bladder channels are also used as they traverse the area of genitals.

Irregular menstruation	Du. 20, Ren. 4, Ren. 6, U.B. 23, U.B. 32, Sp. 6, K. 3
Painful periods	Du. 20, Ren. 3, Ren. 4, Ren. 6, U.B. 32, L.I. 4, St. 44, Sp. 6
Excessive bleeding	Du. 20, Ren. 6, Ren. 3, K. 3, Sp. 6, Lu. 9
White discharge	Ren. 2, Ren. 3, G.B. 26, L.I. 11, Sp. 6
Pelvic inflammation	Du. 20, Ren. 4, St. 29, U.B. 32, L.I. 11, U.B. 28, Sp. 6

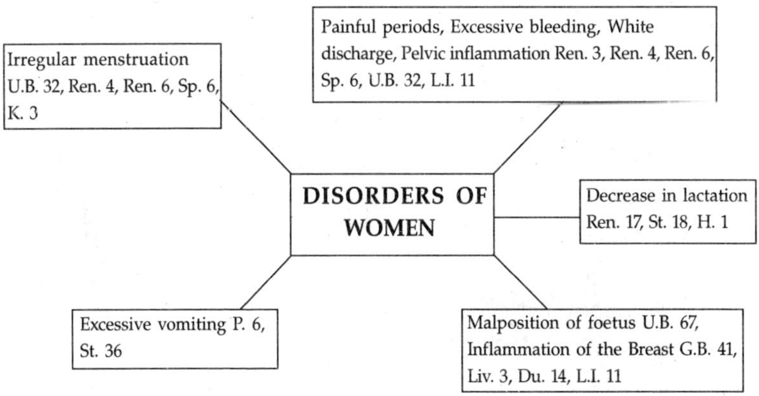

Excessive vomiting	P. 6, St. 36
Malposition of foetus	U.B. 67
For painless delivery	Du. 20, L.I. 4, Sp. 6
Delay of delivery	L.I. 4, Sp. 6, Liv. 3 U.B. 22, G.B. 34
Decrease in lactation	Ren. 17, Sp. 18, H. 1
Inflammation of the breast (due to stagnation of milk during lactation)	S.I. 1, Liv. 3, G.B. 41, Du. 14, L.I. 11

Disorders of Women

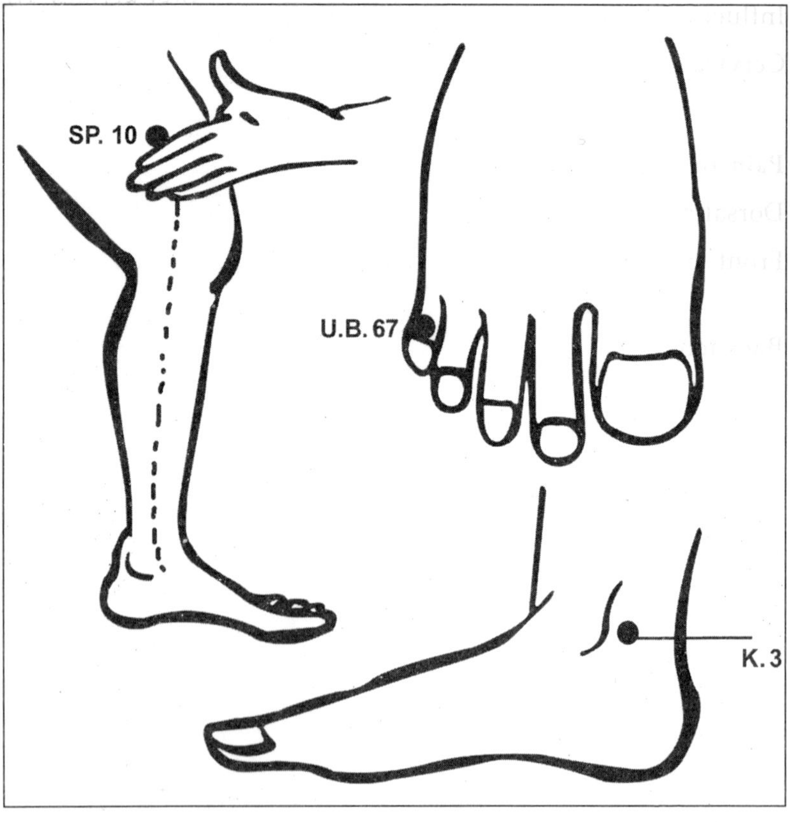

Locomotor Disorders (Diseases of Muscles and Bones)

Important points	—
Analgesic points	L.I. 4, St. 44
Homoeostatic points	L.I. 11, St. 36, Sp. 6
Sedative points	H. 7, U.B. 62, Du. 20
Bone and cartilage Influential point	U.B. 11
Muscle and tendon Influential point	G.B. 34
Cervical spondylosis	Du. 20, U.B. 11, G.B. 20, Du. 14, Lu. 7

Pain in the Chest Region

Dorsal side	Du. 20, U.B. 11, L.I. 4, T.H. 8, Ex. 21
Front side	Du. 20, Liv. 14, G.B. 24, Lu. 1, St. 18, L.I. 4, P. 6
Backache	Du. 20, U.B. parts in the back which are painful U.B. 40, U.B. 60, U.B. 11

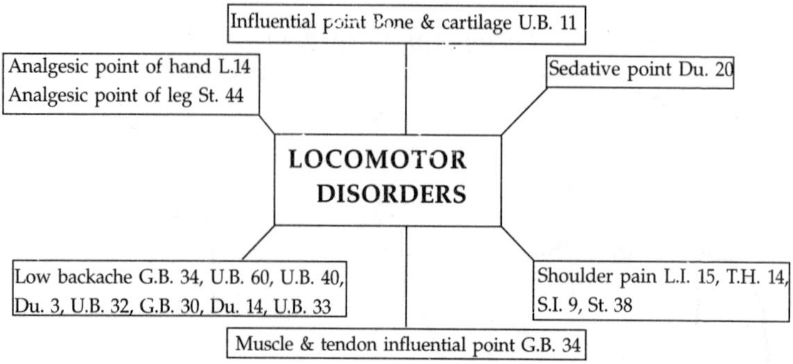

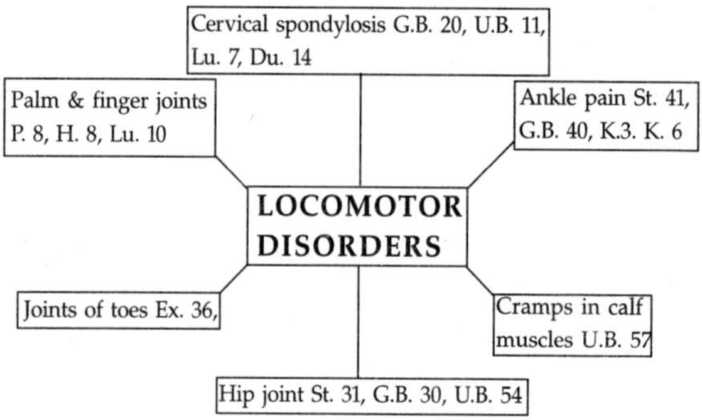

Low backache	Du. 20, Du. 3, Du. 4, U.B. 32, U.B. 33, U.B. 40, U.B. 60, G.B. 30, T.H. 8, G.B. 34
Shoulder pain (frozen shoulder)	Du. 20, L.I. 15, T.H. 14, S.I. 9, L.I. 4, St. 38, G.B. 34
Elbow pain (tennis elbow)	Lu. 5, P. 3, H. 7, L.I. 11, L.I. 4
Wrist pain	Du. 20, P. 7, H. 7, Lu. 9, Lu. 7, L.I. 4, G.B. 34
Palm and finger joints	Du. 20, Lu. 10, P. 8, H. 8, L.I. 4
Hip joint	G.B. 30, U.B. 54, U.B. 32, St. 31, L.I. 4.

Locomotor Disorders

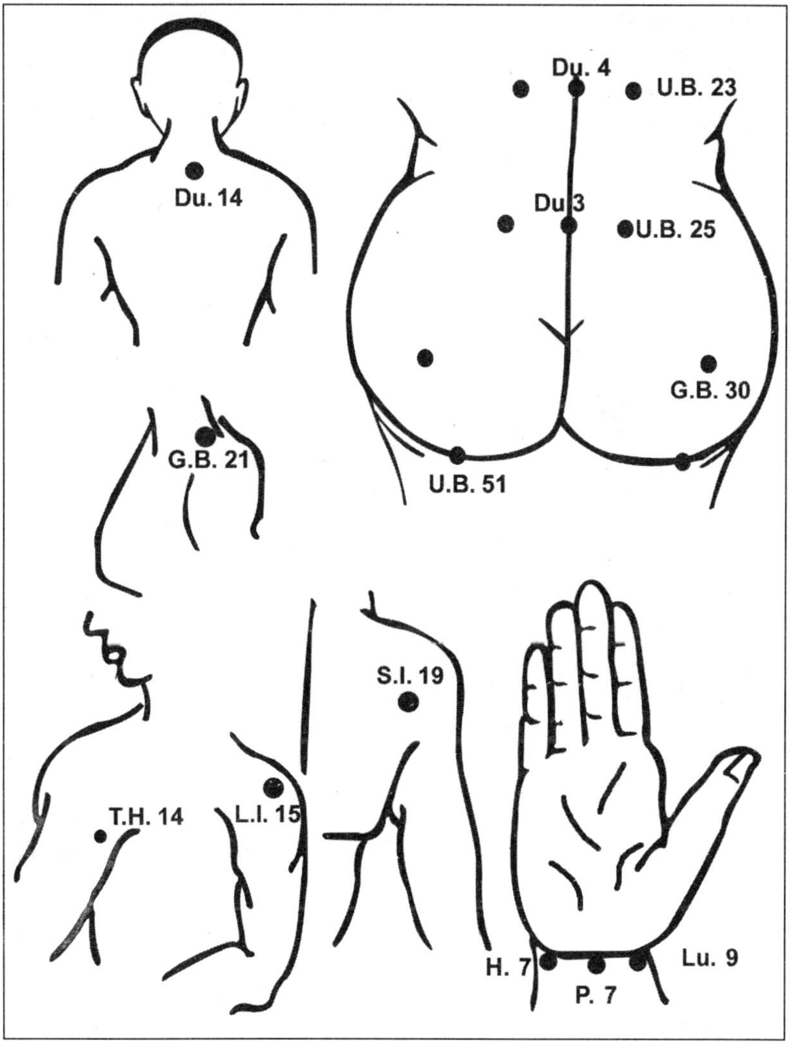

Knee joint	Du. 20, Ex. 35, St. 36, Sp. 10, U.B. 40, L.I. 4, U.B. 11, Sp. 9
Ankle pain	Du. 20, K. 3, K. 6, St. 41, G.B. 40, L.I. 4
Foot pain	Du. 20, St. 44, L.I. 4

Sole of the foot	Du. 20, K. 3, K. 1, L.I. 4
Joint of toes	Du. 20, Ex. 36, L.I. 4
Cramps in calf muscles	U.B. 57
Warts	K.1, K. 3, L.I. 4

Skin Disorders

Important Points

Lung channel		Lu. 5, Lu. 9 (for the skin & vascular system)
Kidney channel		K. 3, K. 10 (for baldness & grey hair)
Du. Channel	Immune enhancing	Du. 14
	sedative	Du. 20
Large intestine	Homoeostatic	L.I. 11

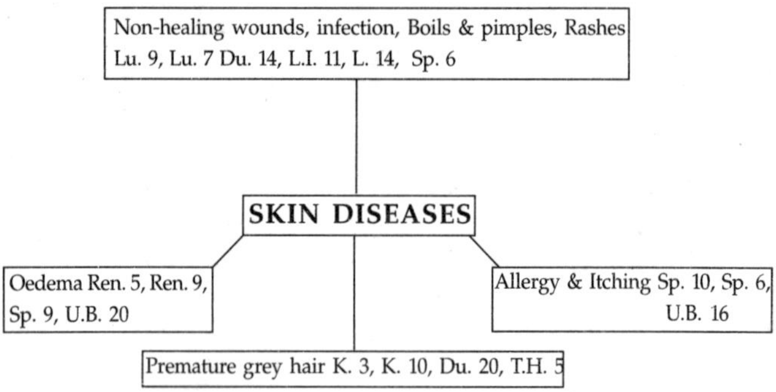

Non-healing wounds and ulcers of the skin	Du. 20, Lu. 9, Lu. 7 & local points on the opposite of the lesion
For infection, allergy & itching	Du. 14, L.I. 11, Sp. 10, U.B. 16

Boils & pimples	Du. 20, L.I. 4 (if in face), Lu. 5, Lu. 7
Warts	Du. 20, Lu. 7, Local points. Du. 14 (Immune enhancing) L.I. 11
Anti-allergic	Sp. 6, Sp. 10
Rashes	Du. 20, Sp. 10, L.I. 11, Du. 14, Lu. 5, Sp. 6, St. 36
Severe cases	H. 6, H. 7, P. 6, U.B. 15 U.B. 62, U.B. 16 (for itching)
Elephantiasis	Du. 20, Ren. 9, Ren. 5, Sp. 9, U.B. 20 (for oedema), Du. 14, L.I. 11

Skin Disorders

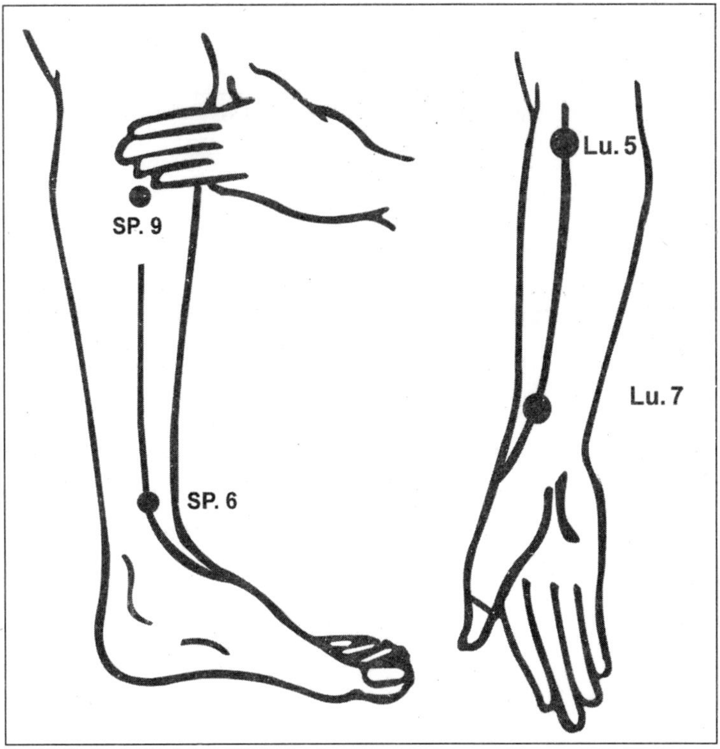

	(immune enhancing), Sp. 6 (allergy)
Herpes	Du. 20, painful points along the affected area, Ex. 21 points adjacent to spinal cord, all Du. points on the spinal column L.I. 4, T.H. 5, T.H. 8, St. 44
Leucoderma	Du. 14, Lu. 7, Sp. 10, L.I. 11, Sp. 6, points close to the affected area.
Sudden bald patches	Du. 20, Ex. 6, Lu. 7, K. 3, K. 10, Lu. 4, T.H. 5
Premature grey hair	K. 3, K. 10, Du. 20.

Ear Disorders

Triple heater, gall bladder, small intestine channels are generally

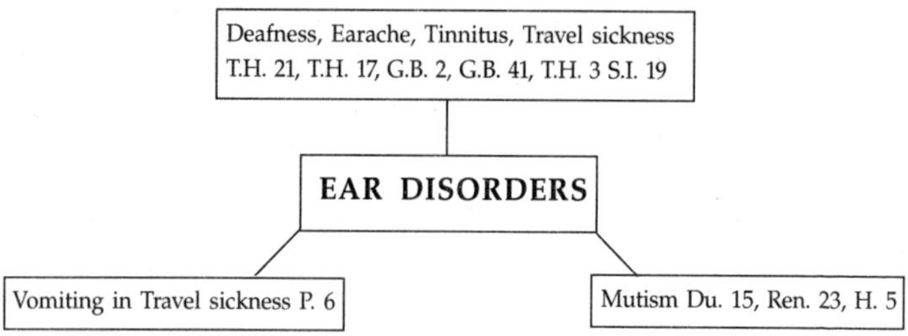

used, whose course traverses near the ear. Kidney channel is also used as kidney is related to ear.

Proximal points close to the ear	T.H. 21, T.H. 17, G.B. 2, S.I. 19
Deafness	Du. 20, T.H. 21, T.H. 19, G.B. 2, T.H. 17, T.H. 3, G.B. 41
Mutism	Du. 15, Ren. 23, H. 5
Tinnitus (ringing in the ears)	Same as deafness.

Ear Disorders

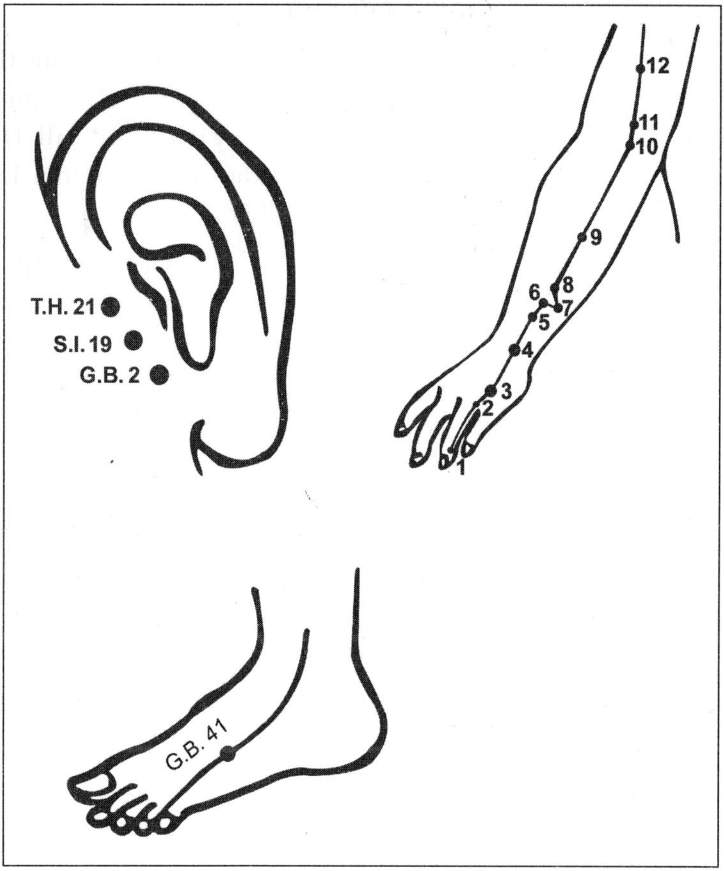

Earache	Same points plus Immune enhancing points Du. 14, L.I. 11, Sp. 6
Travel sickness, vertigo, deafness accompanied by giddiness	All points for deafness plus P. 6 & St. 36 for nausea, vomiting during travel sickness.

Eye Disorders

Important points	
special sense organ point	L.I. 4
Liver channel	Liver opens to the eye. Liv. 3

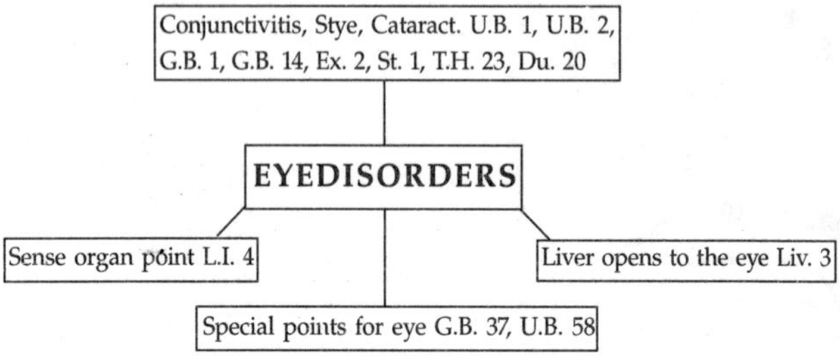

Gall bladder and Urimary bladder channel	U.B. 18, connected to liver. U.B. 19, connected to G.B.
Special points	G.B. 37, U.B. 58
Proximal points to the eye	U.B. 1, U.B. 2, Ex. 1, Ex. 2, Ex. 3, St. 1, T.H. 23, St. 1, G.B. 1, G.B. 20
Conjunctivitis	Du. 20, Ex. 2, U.B. 1, T.H. 23, St. 1, G.B. 1, G.B. 20.
Stye	Du. 20, Ex. 3, T.H. 23, U.B. 1, G.B. 37, Liv. 3, L.I. 4
Detached retina	Du. 20, St. 1, U.B. 2, G.B. 14, G.B. 20, Ex. 2, U.B. 18
Homoeostatic points	L.I. 11, St. 36
Cataract	Du. 20, St. 1, Ex. 2, G.B. 14, U.B. 2, Liv. 3, L.I. 4
Glaucoma	Du. 20, St. 1, Ex. 2, G.B. 14, U.B. 2,

Eye Disorders

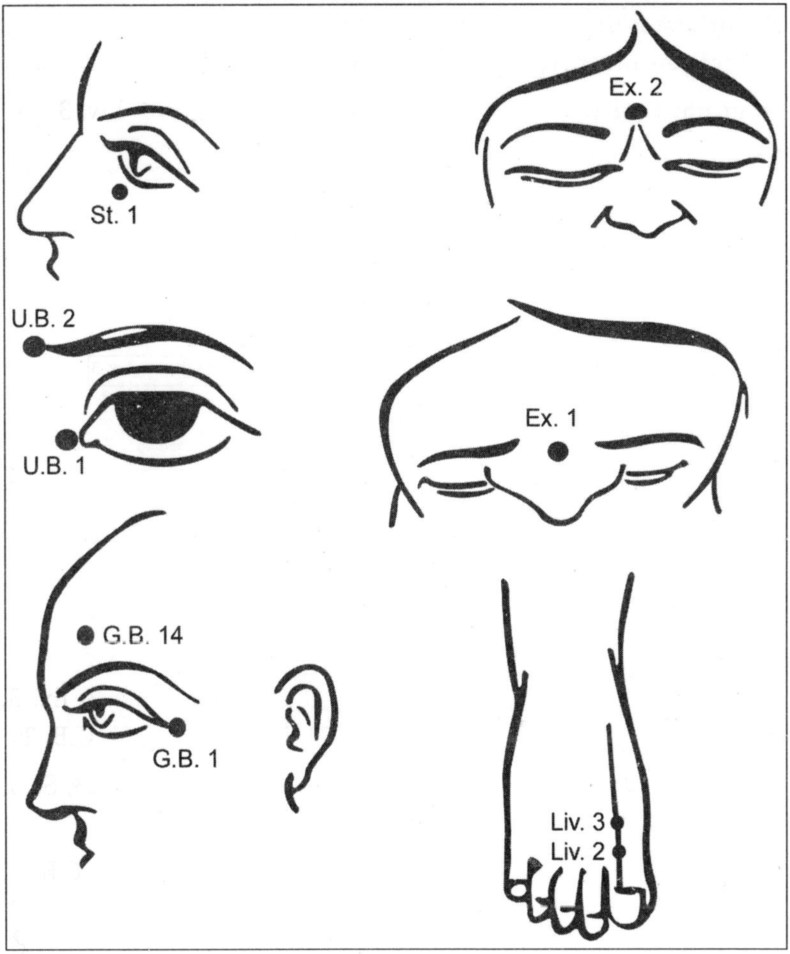

(increase in fluid in the eye ball)	G.B. 20, U.B. 18, Liv. 3, Liv. 4, (Sp. 9, Ren. 6, Ren. 9, for oedema)
Night blindness	Du. 20, St. 1, G.B. 14, U.B. 2, Ex. 2, L.I. 4, G.B. 37, St. 36, Liv. 3

Endocrine Disorders

It includes activities of hypothalamus, pituitary, adrenal, pancreas and other endocrine functions.

Important points

Endocrine points	G.B. 21, T.H. 20, L.I. 18
Homoeostatic and tonification functions	St. 36, Sp. 6, Ren. 6, L.I. 11
Ren. channel	Ren. 2, Ren. 3, Ren. 4, Ren. 6
Kidney channel	K. 3
U.B. channel	U.B. 32, U.B. 33, U.B. 34
Less fertility, decrease	Du. 20, Ren. 2, Ren. 3, St. 29, Ren. 4,
in sperm count, less	K.3 Tonification points, Ren. 6,
libido, secondary sexual characteristic like less facial hair, pubic hair, etc.	St. 36, Sp. 6
Masculine symptoms	Du. 20, Ren. 2, Ren. 3, Ren. 4, Ren. 6,
in women	St. 29, U.B. 32, U.B. 33, U.B. 34, K. 3 Homoeostatic pts. L.I. 11, St. 36, Sp. 6
Goitre	Du. 20, L.I. 18, G.B. 21, L.I. 4
Diabetes	**DU. 20**
Endocrine points	**T.H. 20, L.I. 18, G.B. 21**
Homoeostatic points	**L.I. 11, Sp. 6, St. 36, Liv. 3 & Liv. 13**

Endocrine Disorders

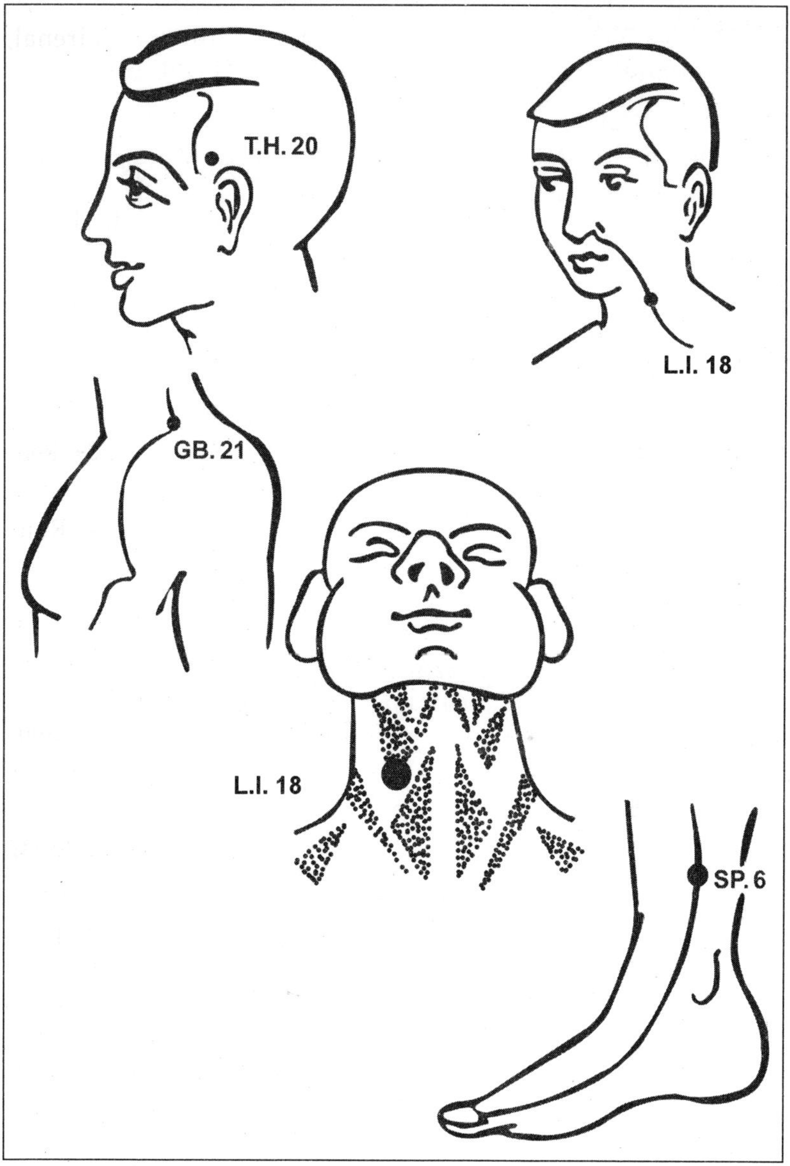

Psychiatric Disorders

Important points

Sedative points	Du. 20, H. 7, U.B. 62
Homoeostatic points	St. 36, Sp. 6, Ren. 6

Du channel, heart and pericardium channels are commonly used. Heart and pericardium are connected to the brain.

Neurosis — Symptoms

Nervousness, irritability, anxiety, depression, insomnia, headache, sexual disorders	Sedative Pts. Du. 20, H. 7, U.B. 62, Ex. 7, Ex. 8, G.B. 20, Sp. 6, Ren. 2, Ren. 4, P. 4
Hysteria	Sedative Pts. Du. 20, H. 7, U.B. 62, Emergency Pts. Du. 26, K. 1, plus P. 6, P. 4, T.H. 5

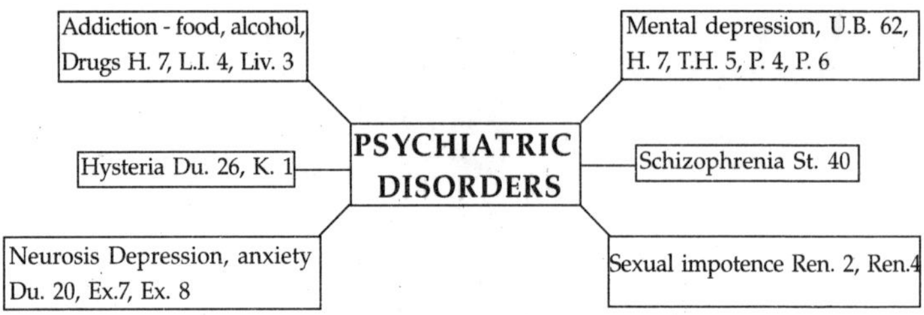

Schizophrenia	Sedative Pts. Du. 20, H. 7, U.B. 62, Du. 26, Du. 14, Ex. 8, Ex. 9, U.B. 15, St. 40, L.I. 4
Mental depression	Sedative Pts. Du. 20, H. 7, U.B. 62, Tonification Pts. St. 36, Sp. 6, Ren. 6
Sexual impotence	Du. 20, Ren. 2, Ren. 3, Ren. 4, Ren. 6, Du. 14, U.B. 23, K. 3, Sp. 6, St. 36
Addiction (drugs, food, alcohol, smoking, betel chewing)	Du. 20, H.7, T.H. 5, Liv. 3, L.I. 4

Psychiatric Disorders

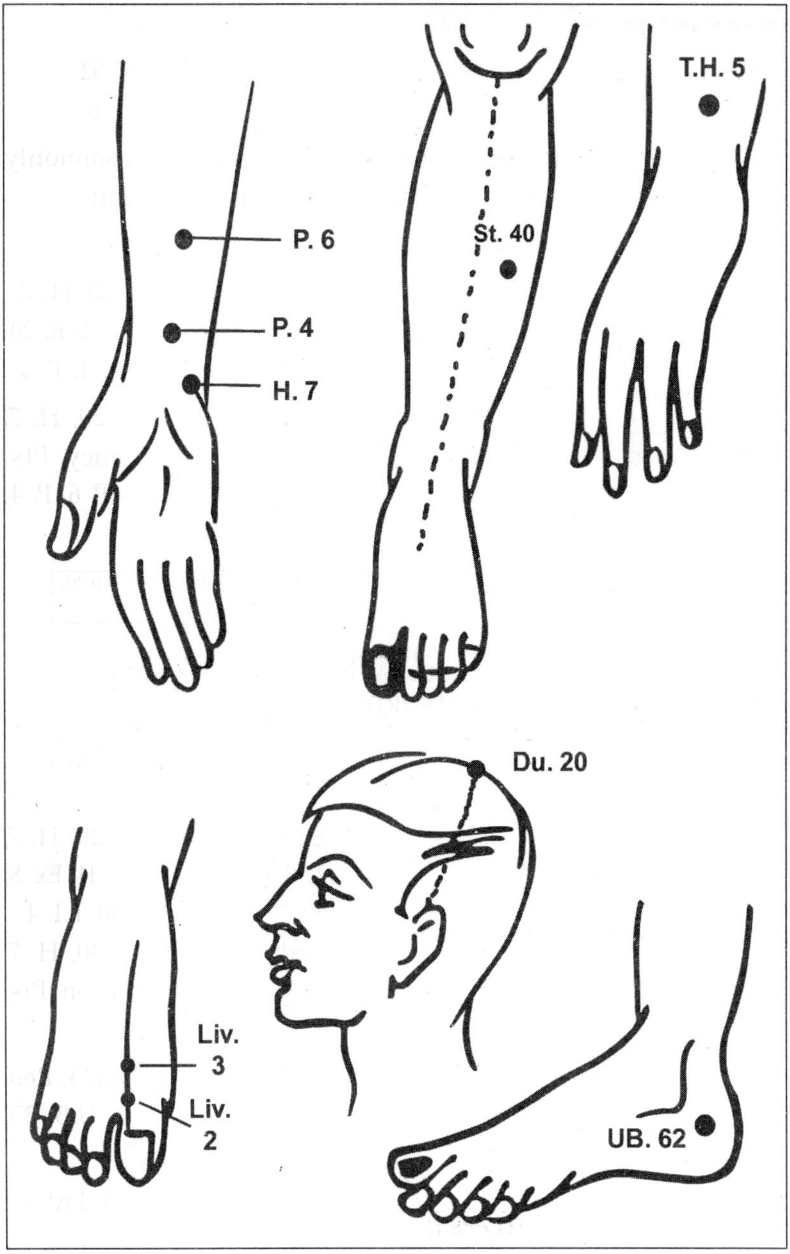

Nervous System Disorders

Important points

Sedative points H. 7, U.B. 62, Du. 20, G.B. 34
(Imp. for nervous debility)

Motor points close to the affected area. Gall bladder, urinary bladder, and Du channel as it traverses the brain.

Epilepsy

Sedative points	H. 7, U.B. 62, Du. 20, Plus Ex. 6
Emergency points	Du. 26
Other points	Ex. 1, Ex. 8, Ex. 9, U.B. 15, G.B. 34, L.I. 4
For excessive sputum	St. 40

Parkinsonism — Symptom — Weakness and spasticity of facial muscle and tremor of hands, excessive salivation, shuffling gait.

Du. 20, Ex. 6, G.B. 34, L.I. 4, St. 44, T.H. 5, H. 7, U.B. 62

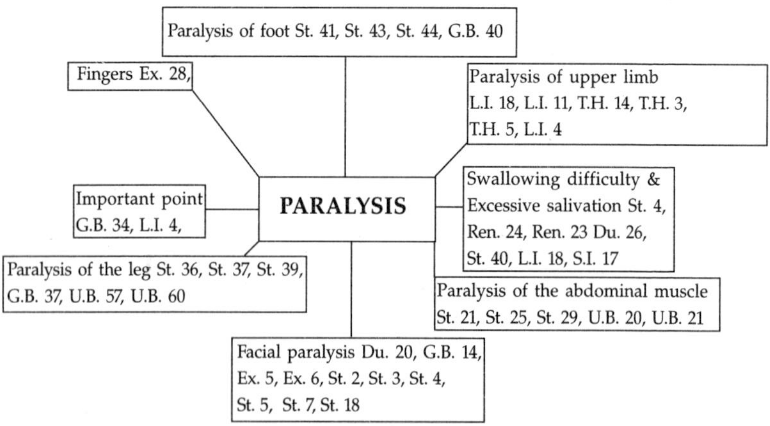

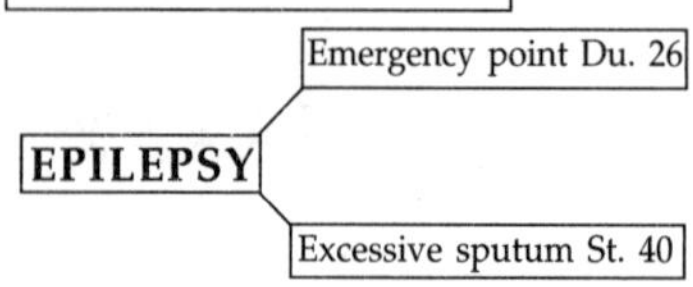

Increased salivation	St. 40, Ren. 23, Ren. 24, St. 4
Headache	Imp. Points Du. 20, Ex. 6, L.I. 4
Frontal headache	Du. 23, St. 8, G.B. 14 (forehead area) Ex. 1, Ex. 2
Temporal headache (sides of forehead)	St. 8, G.B. 8, T.H. 23
Occipital headache (back of the head)	Lu. 7, G.B. 20, U.B. 60
Vertical headache	Liv. 2, U.B. 60, Du. 2
Insomnia	Du. 20, Ex. 8, Ex. 9, H. 7, U.B. 62, P. 6, K. 3, Ex. 6
Meningitis	(inflammation of covering of brain and spinal cord)
	Du. 20, Du. 14, L.I. 11, L.I. 4, St. 36, Ex. 6, U.B. 37, U.B. 60, Sp. 6, U.B. 40, P. 6
Paralysis	Imp. Points Du. 20, Ex. 6, G.B. 34
Facial paralysis	Du. 20, Ex. 6, G.B. 14, Ex. 2, St. 2, St. 3, St. 4, St. 5, St. 7, St. 18, L.I. 4, G.B. 34

Paralysis of the body

Upper limb (arm)	L.I. 15, L.I. 11, T.H. 14, T.H. 3, T.H. 5, L.I. 4
Fingers	Ex. 28
Leg (thigh)	St. 31, St. 32, G.B. 30, G.B. 31
Lower leg	St. 36, St. 37, St. 39, G.B. 37, U.B. 57, U.B. 60
Foot	St. 41, St. 43, St. 44, G.B. 40.
Swallowing difficulty	Ren. 23, Ren. 24, P. 6, Du. 26, L.I. 18, L.I. 4, S.I. 17

Nervous System Disorders

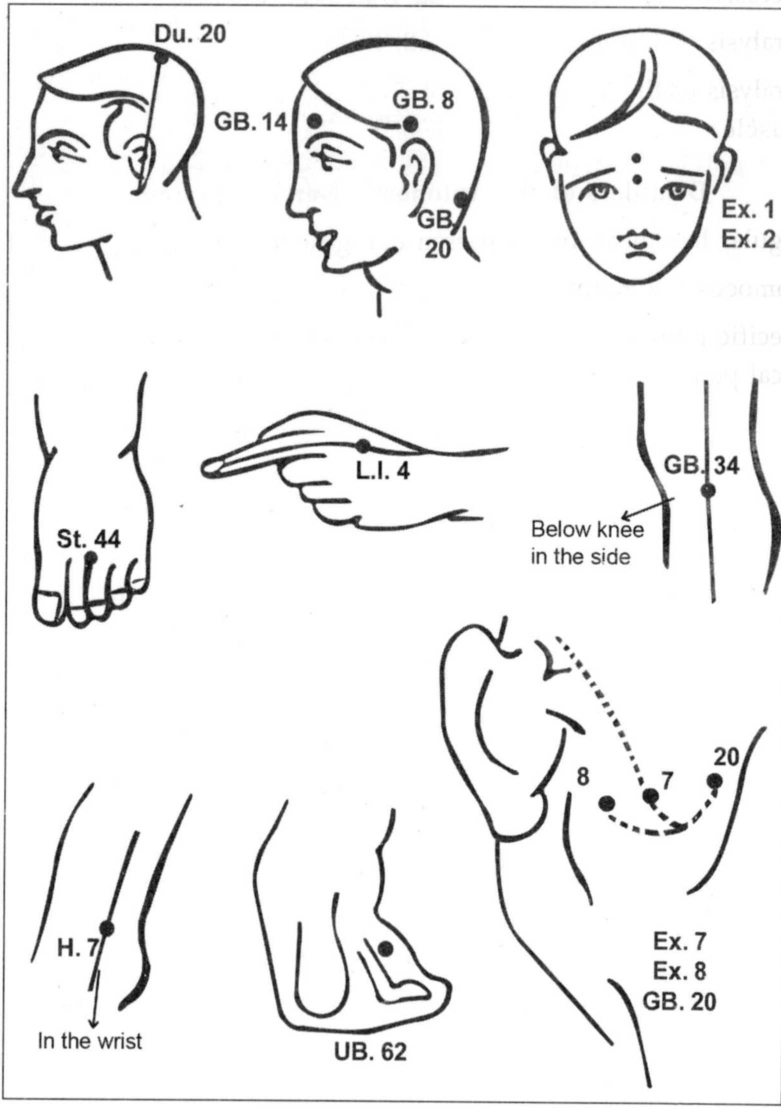

Excessive salivation	St. 4, Ren. 24, Ren. 23, St. 40
Paralysis of the diaphragm	U.B. 17, Liv. 14
Paralysis of the abdominal Muscle	St. 21, St. 25, St. 29, U.B. 20 U.B. 21

Disorders of the Autonomic Nervous System

Regular heartbeat, blood pressure, digestive activities.

Homoeostatic points	L.I. 11, St. 36, Sp. 6
Specific points	H. 6, H. 7, L.I. 4

Local points as per affliction

11

Extra Points

THERE are some extra points apart from the channel points.

The important ones are Ex. 1, Ex. 2, Ex. 6, Ex. 7, Ex. 8, Ex. 33 and Ex. 32.

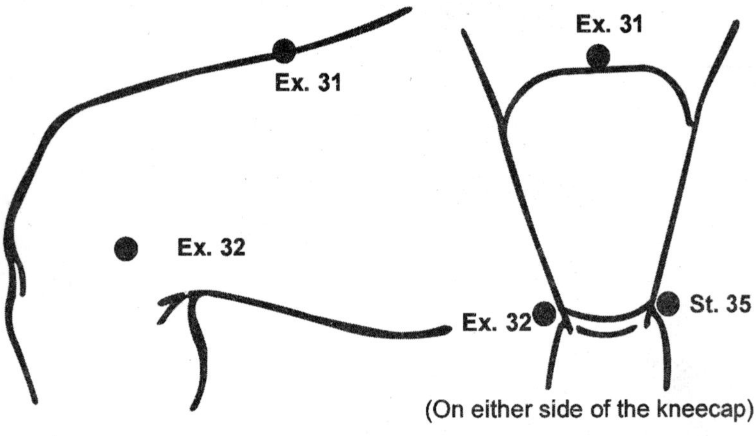

Ex. 31 on the mid pt. above the upper border of the kneecap.
– Disorders of knee joint.

Ex. 32 Along the inner side of the kneecap, in the depression.
– Disorders of knee joint.

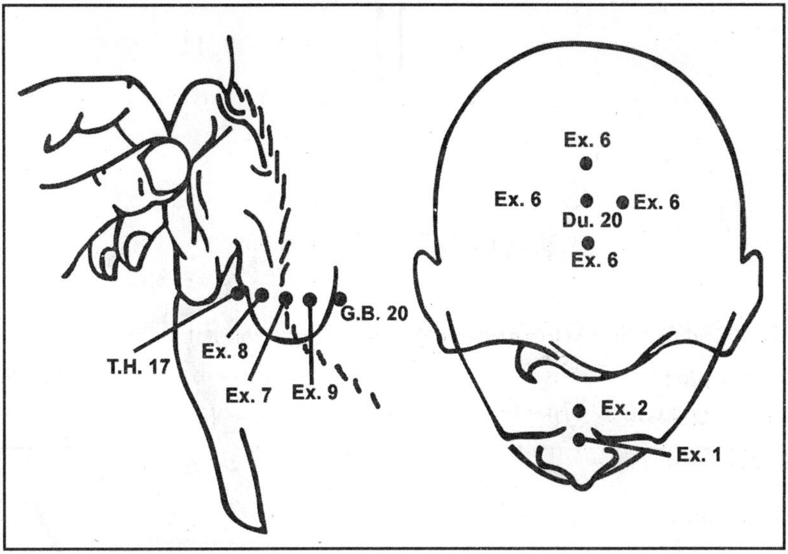

Ex. 6 : On the Vortex of the head
1 chun anterior, postenor and lateral to DU. 20.
Helps in heavy headache, epilepsy

Ex. 7 : 1 chun laternal to T.H. 17
Ear and eye disorders, insomnia

Ex. 8 : Between T.H. 17 and Ex. 7
Ear and eye disorders, insomnia.

Ex.9 : Between Ex. 7 and G.B. 20
Insomnia.

12

Kundalini Energy

To associate Kundalini energy with acupressure

1st Chakra

Mooladhara chakra (earth energy)	—	Du. 2	Adrenal

2nd Chakra

Swadishthana (water energy)	—	Du. 4	Reproductive Glands

3rd Chakra

Manipoora (fire energy)	—	Du. 6	Solar Plexus, Pancreas

4th Chakra

Anahata (air energy)	—	Du. 11	Heart & Thymus

5th Chakra

Vishuddha (ether energy)	—	Du. 14	Throat & Thyroid

6th Chakra

Ajna (Mental energy)	—	Du. 16	Pituitary

7th Chakra

Sahasrara (Samadhi)	—	Du. 20	

13

Important Instructions for the Practitioner

1. Acupressure points are very tiny spot-like points. If the points are not properly located and acted upon, the treatment does not give the desired effect. These points are just below the skin so they can be easily located by pinching at that place. Once the point is located, pressure can be applied by the use of thumb, fingers, or a blunt stick like non-writing end of a ballpen.
2. Do not apply acupressure either on empty stomach or immediately after intake of food.
3. Generally pressure can be applied on a particular point for the duration of 10 seconds to 2 minutes.
4. Pressure should be applied in proportion to the individual capacity of tolerance of each patient. Applying too much of pressure may harm, instead of benefiting the patient.
5. Males, females, children, young men and elderly people have different levels of tolerance. Therefore the duration and the intensity of pressure applied must also be different in each case.
6. Acupressure treatment is generally given once a day. But in special cases, if necessary the treatment can be repeated twice or thrice a day. Similarly if the patient is unable to bear the treatment daily, he can be given the treatment on alternate days.

7. Pressure must not be applied on the points on the stomach or the back of a pregnant woman. On the points on other parts of the body too, pressure must be applied only lightly especially in the case of young children or the elderly.
8. In case of too much fatigue and in case of surgeries, light pressure must be applied very carefully avoiding the areas operated upon or area that are extremely painful.
9. At times, while taking acupressure treatment on one hand, people continue with their old harmful food and work habits on the other. This only hampers the treatment. In order to draw the maximum benefits from acupressure treatment, it will be conducive to the treatment if along with taking the treatment one must carefully avoid eating too much or too little, leading an extremely busy or sedentary life, being too emotional, depressive, negative attitude to life, etc. becuase all these are very harmful for health and will work against the treatment.

14

Case Histories

ACUPRESSURE/ACUPUNCTURE is an excellent and effective form of treatment in most of the painful disorders. Due to its efficacy and lack of side effects it should be advocated as the first line of treatment in the problems of osteoarthritis, rheumatoid arthritis, migraine, neurological pain, etc.

As this science works at the energy level and through the energy meridians, **it has direct access to each of the vital organs like liver, spleen, kidney, heart and lungs.** It acts as a rejuvenating mechanism vitalising the organs and in turn attending to the root of the disease by organ correction. Thus problems ranging from common cold to chronic asthma, gets instant relief with just few sittings of accupuncture/acupressure.

This aspect makes it useful practically for all health problems, since most of them stem from organ impairment. Except for mechanical problems like fracture or accident, most of the physiological, pathological and even psychological health problems can be effectively treated under this discipline.

Few of the divergent health problems dealt with are discussed below:

1. Frozen shoulder
2. Low backache
3. Acute knee pain
4. Heel pain
5. Trigeminal neuralgia
6. Rheumatoid arthritis
7. Hearing problem
8. Epilepsy
9. Chronic headache
10. Wheezing and asthma

11. Bells palsy — Facial paralysis
12. Insomnia and depression
13. Falling hair
14. Swelling in the body
15. Pox marks on face

1. Frozen Shoulder

A 52-year-old lady Damayanti Desai found suddenly she could not raise her right hand above her neck, neither she could take it back to comb her hair nor wear her saree with ease. When she arrived to acupuncture clinic the problem was four months old. Many other treatments had been tried.

I inserted a needle at L.I. 4, the relief was instantaneous, further needling at St. 38 (opp. side), G.B. 34, T.H. 5, improved the situation. In all it took only four treatments to give her complete cure.

2. Low Backache

Many cases of low backache are routinely treated by acupuncture with good results. On an average backache responds by 10 to 15 sittings admirably. There are cases of dramatic recovery too.

U.B. 23, U.B. 25, Du. 3, Du. 4, K. 3, Sp. 6 are some of the points routinely used.

3. Acute Knee Pain

Mrs. Bharti Rathod is a 42-year-old school teacher with a heavy build. She brought her X-ray which showed her right knee joint bereft of the protective cartilage and degenerative process had set in the bones. She was getting acute pain while climbing stairs and while bending. She was advised knee replacement. She took two and a half month treatment. The improvement was gradual but steady. At the end of the treatment her pain was almost gone. After checking the doctors opined the operation can be avoided.

U.B. 11, K. 3, K. 7 and local points were used for treatment.

4. Heel Pain

Mrs. Geeta Venkatesh, an active lady of 40 years, found her right heel is subjected to acute pin prick like pain, more so in the morning for first one hour of getting out of bed. The pain was almost intolerable to carry out her daily routine. After 15 days of the pain she came to acupuncture treatment. After administration of five sitting of treatment she experienced complete relief.

Pts applied were U.B. 62, K. 3, K. 5, U.B. 11. Ear pts. were also electronically stimulated.

5. Trigeminal Neuralgia

Mrs. L.N. Shah was a young man in his 30s and computer engineer by profession. He started getting shooting pain from the left cheek to the temple. Drastic use of painkillers gave him relief for short period only. He was advised tooth extraction and had two of his molars removed. He came for treatment 3 months after the problem started.

Treatment was started on the opposite side of the face. Recovery was swift. His face started visibly relaxing after third treatment. He completed the course of 15 treatments to avoid any recurrence.

Pts. used: H. 1, P. 6, Du. 20, S.I. 18, St. 3, S.I. 6, St. 7, etc.

6. Rheumatoid Arthritis

Sixty-year-old Padmavati Purandhare was suffering from deforming rheumatoid arthritis for more than 15 years. She had a history of tuberculosis of spine 10 years before. She was subjected to heavy medication. She was at the time of treatment bedridden with right leg completely stiff, had poor appetite and typical case of polyarthritis.

Treatment was carried out for 3 months continuously. First by using balancing and immune enhancing points (St. 36, Liv. 11, Sp. 6) her appetite and sleep was restored, further onslaught of the disease was checked. Her right leg stiffness was eased and she started walking around the house. Her kidney working was improved which made her buoyant and almost normal. Her deformation was corrected only partially. However, she was able to carry out normal activity in spite of the deformation.

For all kinds of arthritis, acupuncture should be advised with-out fail to arrest the disease and make the pain tolerable.

7. Hearing Problem

Miss Shilpa Nair, a young college girl, developed sudden hearing loss at the age of eighteen after administration of a drug for ear pain and puss. Her hearing loss was detected at the range of 75db. She was also getting occasional ringing in the ears. The family was totally shaken. She was brought to acupuncture after nearly a year when she had a hearing aid attached to her ear.

It was a case of nerve deafness. Two sets of treatment having 20 sittings in each were given to her. Both local points and kidney points were tonified as kidney governs hearing. Her hearing loss came to 30db and she was able to work without hearing aid.

A further course of 15 sittings removed the problem completely.

8. Epilepsy

Acupuncture is a safe and sure answer to many suffering from epilepsy and who have to be under constant medication throughout life.

A number of epileptic cases have been treated successfully. The medicine is tapered gradually. In six months to one year even severe cases can live without medication and epileptic fits fully under control.

Pts. used: Du. 20, Ex. 6, H. 7, P. 6, Ex. 1.

9. Chronic Headache

Mrs. Malini Kapoor aged 32 years was a typical case of chronic headache which had precipitated into migraine attacks with passage of time. Married with a 7-year-old child and a busy office schedule had heightened her problem. She could spare only the weekend for treatment.

Two sittings were given to her every week. In four months of treatment her headache vanished completely and she started looking fresh and relaxed.

Pts. Du. 20, Ex. 6, St. 8, G.B. 14, L.I. 4, St. 44.

10. Wheezing and Asthma

Haribhai Patel, at 55 was heavy set, panting for breath constantly and had a history of 20 years of asthma. His bronchioles on examination were found inflamed and constricted. He had stock of all emergency medicines constantly with him.

His case was one of the lung excess often found in asthma. His lung energy was sedated, kidney was improved to bring about cooling. Ear points of lung and asthma treated. Ear press needle was administered. His attacks started reducing, in six months' time he showed good improvement and started leading normal life.

11. Bells Palsy — Facial Paralysis

Naren Upadhyaya at the age of 44 was a travelling sales person. After a bus ride on a particularly cold winter night with a defective window of the bus kept open, he had an attack of bells palsy with part of his face becoming paralytic. Luckily he was soon brought for acupuncture treatment. It took just 4 treatments to bring him back to normal.

Pts. used: Local points, G.B. 34, L.I. 4, St. 44.

Both partial paralysis like bells palsy and total paralysis generally after stroke respond very well under acupuncture treatment.

Any nerve related problem including polio, even after a lapse of many years respond to acupuncture much better in comparison to drug therapy as the impulses are passed directly to the nerves by body and scalp acupuncture.

12. Insomnia and Depression

Mrs. Meera Jetli at the age of 47 years was going through her menopause. Her children had left home. The hormone changes and situation in life gave her bout of depression and sleepless nights for 6 months in a row. She had developed dark circles under the eyes and her skin was loose and cracked showing yin dryness.

A set of 10 sittings administered to her turned to be a great tonic for her. Sedative points (Du. 20, H. 7) brought her anxiety down. She started getting fitful sleep. Improving her kidney and liver working removed the chronic dryness and brought glean to her skin and hope to her life. She developed some interest and started leading more useful life.

Pts. used: K. 3, Liv. 3, Liv. 8, L.I. 11, Du. 14, H. 7.

Many psychiatric problems get very good relief with acupuncture.

13. Falling Hair

A young boy after one-year stay in a hostel for professional studies returned home with near bald scalp. He had total hair loss in the front. His hair was coming out in tufts. His skin was pale and he was feeling difficult and shy to face the world.

An intense treatment of fifteen sittings was administered during his holidays. It was hard to believe for him, the lost hair started coming out short and thick. In a month's time his scalp was filled with hair.

Both his lung and kidney working was improved. His chronic constipation was rectified.

Pts. used: Lu. 9, Lu. 7, L.I. 4, K. 3, K. 7 and local points.

14. Swelling in the Body

Mrs. Sheetal Vyas developed oedema in both her legs, her abdomen also was bloated. The development was gradual after she suffered from severe malaria 6 months back. Urine increasing drugs reduced her swelling overnight only to get it back again. She was given acupuncture for one month. After four sittings only she showed good improvement. The oedema started waning. The pale parlour of her skin was getting healthy.

Her spleen, liver, kidney improved in the working. Ren. points were treated with needling and moxa. Her oedema disappeared and she was back to good health.

Pts. Used: St. 36, Sp. 6, L.I. 11, Sp. 9, Ren. 6, Ren. 9.

15. Pox Marks on the Face

For 22-year-old Vinya, a bright girl with an MBA degree, the pox marks left by childhood chicken pox were a big drag. She did not want to go for plastic surgery, skin lotions were not getting her anywhere. She decided to try acupuncture. She was given treatment in stomach meridian and sedative points administered as she was very hyper with activity. The results were quite good. Her colleagues commented on decrease in pox marks and her glowing complexion. She also started getting fitful sleep.